The User's Guide to the Male Body

JIM POLLARD

To everyone past and present at the Men's Health Forum

First published in Great Britain in 2009

Sheldon Press
36 Causton Street
London SW1P 4ST

British Library Cataloguing-in-Publication Data
A catalogue record for this book is available from the British Library

ISBN 978–1–84709–042–3

1 3 5 7 9 10 8 6 4 2

Typeset by Fakenham Photosetting Ltd, Fakenham, Norfolk
Printed in Great Britain by Ashford Colour Press

Produced on paper from sustainable forests

Contents

About the author   v

Foreword   vii

Acknowledgements   viii

Introduction   ix

   The book you should have been born with   ix

1 The basics   1

   How long have you got?   1

   Why you should risk reading on   9

2 The key applications inside out   12

   The brain   12

   The heart   16

   The penis and testicles   20

   The prostate   28

   Networking with other systems: the ins and outs of sex   30

3 Beyond the basics: the lazy man's troubleshooting guide   36

   Eating: want weight loss without great loss?   37

   Alcohol: when does serious drinking become dangerous
drinking?   46

   Exercise: want to get back in the game?   52

   Work: the twenty-first century's biggest threat to health?   63

   Addiction: how can something that felt so good feel
so bad?   71

   Depression: as dangerous as smoking?   77

   Mid-life crisis: the best thing that ever happened to you?   85

4 When the system goes down: how to be ill with skill   89

   What do I do when I'm ill?   89

   How do I talk about the thing I can't talk about?   97

   How do I handle a health problem?   100

5 Inside the operating system: A–Z of other user-
   serviceable parts   107

6 DIY health check   125

7 A little summary   128

Useful addresses   129

Further reading   131

Index   133

About the author

Jim Pollard is editor of the award-winning website <malehealth.co.uk>. Run by the Men's Health Forum, it is the only website in the world that provides a free, comprehensive, independent health information service for men by men. Formerly health editor of Maxim magazine and a health columnist and writer in both tabloid and broadsheet newspapers, he was recently shortlisted for the Patients' Association health journalist of the year award.

Jim is the author of six health books, including the acclaimed All Right, Mate? and a novel. Among his various health adventures, he had lymphatic cancer in the 1990s and as a result has enjoyed radiotherapy, chemotherapy and many of the other fun-packed procedures that a man can be called on to endure in the name of his health.

His personal website is <jimpollard.co.uk>.

Foreword

When all else fails, read the instruction manual.

There is no shortage of advice for men – a great deal of it but little of it great. Unfortunately, most of the stuff out there is patronizing, stereotypical, badly informed, poorly researched or more often all four.

Jim Pollard is a true men's health expert. Not only has he experienced serious ill health to focus his mind on the shortcomings of our health services, but he is also actively involved in the men's health arena, giving a great part of his life to promoting male health. As editor of <malehealth.co.uk> he has ensured its place as the most visited, independent award-winning health site for men in the world. An extension of this hugely popular site, this book takes all the knowledge and experience onto the written page – much easier to read in the bath than a computer and less likely to electrocute.

This no-nonsense book truly reflects men's concerns and, much more importantly, shows men what they can do about them. Risk-taking may be predominantly a male characteristic but this book dramatically shows how to reduce risk by recognizing these behaviours from the outset. It is fun and it ferociously attacks male myths when it comes to health. Like any good instruction manual, it enables men to take control of their own health. At the same time it is gritty and refuses to skirt the issues, instead placing men at the centre of their health care. Go and buy a lads' mag if you are offended by Jim's straight health talk.

This book is timely and will be timeless – not least because it contains common sense as well as high-grade, well-researched advice that men can use. It will save male lives and also have an impact on their partners' and children's health. Jim Pollard has once again confirmed his place as a truly committed 'great' in the newly emerging phenomenon of men's health. Y chromosome owners will never be the same again.

Ian Banks

President of the Men's Health Forum and of the European Men's Health Forum; Professor of European Men's Health, Leeds Metropolitan University; and author of The Man Manual

Acknowledgements

Thanks to fellow men's health authors Ian Banks, Peter Baker and Alan White, and everyone else at the Men's Health Forum for all their help with this book. Thanks also to the members of the various voluntary, statutory and research bodies who answered my questions. Thanks to Bela for her usual stoicism in the face of my unreasonable behaviour over my unreasonable deadlines. And thanks most of all to the many men who have written to the website I edit, <malehealth.co.uk>, where some of this material has previously appeared in a different form. Regardless of whether their stories have appeared on the site or in this book, it is these men's experiences and insights that have informed my writing. All the errors and omissions, on the other hand, are entirely my own.

Introduction

The book you should have been born with

There's no shortage of health advice for men. Mothers are full of it, partners too. The media carries its fair share, and then there are the websites – thousands of them. Some (such as <malehealth.co.uk>, which I edit) are better than others (those that are trying to sell you something). Yes, there's no shortage of health advice, but half of the time it doesn't make sense, often contradicts itself, and working it all out is – for most of us – simply not at the top of our priorities.

What if, like me, you're one of those males who just can't get worked up about the number of portions of veg he has eaten and has better things to do with his time than watch MTV in the gym? That's where this book comes in.

From computers to consoles to cars, most high-tech gadgets these days come *without* a user's manual, and the human body is no exception. You have to work out how to use it by yourself. Fortunately, like the best kit, the body is pretty intuitive. It tends to do what you want it to do most of the time, and common sense will get you a long way when it doesn't.

However, and this it shares with most high-tech gadgets, the human body can easily become old before its time – in the case of the male body *way* before its time. Every year in the UK about 120,000 men die a premature death – that's one young male death every four minutes. The way we use our bodies and how we fuel them can see them beginning to break down decades sooner than necessary, and unlike your new computer you can't just go out and buy a cheaper, more powerful replacement (although your partner might).

The good news is that compared with even the highest-tech products, the human body is far, far better designed and uses a level of technology that geeks can only dream of. Keeping it running smoothly is easy. Anyone can do it. This book explains how.

So what do I know about it? Am I a doctor? No, I was a patient. My body broke down way before its time. I got cancer in my early thirties. At the time I knew very little about health and had to learn quickly. I've been writing about men's health ever since in newspapers and magazines, and most recently as editor of the Men's Health Forum's excellent health information site for men of all ages: <malehealth.co.uk>.

Now, I've nothing against doctors – some of my best friends are doctors (honest! – see Dr Ian Banks' foreword) – but I don't think that medical training provides anything like as much insight into the way we men really think about our health as talking to and interviewing dozens of men about the subject, which is what I've been doing over the past few years. This book is the result.

It explains what you need to know in fewer than 150 pages, with no medical waffle and no visits to the gym (unless you fancy it). In fact, unless they dismantle the NHS (not out of the question, unfortunately), read this book and you shouldn't have to pay a penny more for your health care for many a year. The book focuses on two things:

- prevention – avoiding getting ill in the first place
- what to do when that doesn't work.

The answer to the second one is pretty simple, by the way. Go and see someone. Your GP (general practitioner) is usually the best bet, but there's more on that in Chapter 4.

I haven't tried to go beyond this and tell you all about the various illnesses and diseases you might get and how they're treated. A book with all that detail would be great for dipping into, but let's be honest – you'd probably only read it if you had something specific on your mind. What I've tried to do here is write a book that a man who is *not* feeling ill, who's fit and well, can happily read all the way through.

Once you've read it you'll be armed and ready, able to tell the good from the bad and to surf the health sites of the internet in reasonable safety. It's the book I would have liked to have read before I became ill.

If you want a more comprehensive, all round book on men's health, there are a fair few out there. Some of them aren't very good but three excellent ones are listed in the Further reading section at the end of this book.

1
The basics

This chapter will help you to work out your health risk and what you can do to reduce it.

How long have you got?

Here's an uncomfortable fact. When it comes to premature death, men corner the market. Two out of three deaths before the age of 65 are in men. Every year, 120,000 men – more than the capacity of Wembley stadium, more than the entire British Army – die before they reach the age of 75. It is the equivalent of two Boeing 737s full of men falling from the sky every day. Will you be among them?

I don't know for certain how long you'll live, and neither do you, but you can get a better idea by completing the 'How long have I got?' checklist below. It's not highly scientific – just a bit of fun – but if nothing else it'll help you to decide whether you will be around long enough to take this book back to the library (and, more seriously, just how much of this book you really need to read).

Checklist: How long have I got?

Tick the box (or boxes) next to every statement that applies to you.

Age
- I am over 35 ☐
- I am also over 65 ☐

Inherited health risks
Among my family (including grandparents), there have been two or more cases of:

- heart disease ☐
- cancer ☐
- stroke ☐

- other disease that tends to run in families (e.g. diabetes) □
- suicide □

I have had:
- heart disease □ □
- cancer □ □
- stroke □ □
- other disease that tends to run in families (e.g. diabetes) □ □

Lifestyle
- I smoke □ □ □ □ □
- I drink more than 10 pints or the equivalent a week □
- I binge drink □
- I eat red meat more than a couple of times a week □
- I eat fried food more than a couple of times a week □
- I eat fewer than four portions of fruit and veg a day □
- I have a waist measurement of 37 inches or more □
- I also have a waist measurement of 40 inches or more □
- I exercise fewer than three times a week
  (for 20 minutes at a time) □
- In fact, I never exercise □
- I live in a big city □
- I rarely go out in the sunlight □
- I usually sunbathe without protection □
- I work in a stressful environment over which I have little
  influence □
- I have no job □
- I regularly work more than eight hours a day □
- I don't have a long-term relationship □
- I don't know how to relax □
- I don't take a holiday every year □
- I have sex less than once a week □
- I haven't really got any close friends □

Attitudes
- I work hard and play hard □
- I'm very ambitious □
- I often get angry □
- I worry about what others think of me □
- I find it difficult to talk about how I feel □
- I take life very seriously □

The verdict:
So are you on the way out or on the way up?

- *Over 35* This quiz perhaps arrived a little late for you, but we're glad to see that they're publishing quality non-fiction on the other side.
- *30–34* Stub out that fag, put down the scotch, turn off the telly and read this book.
- *20–29* There are many attractions to old age such as cardigan wearing, dribbling and making outrageous propositions to nurses without fear of a comeback, but you're not going to enjoy any of them unless you give the contents of this book some serious consideration.
- *15–19* You may make it to pensionable age with some serious life-style changes – to begin, read on.
- *10–14* The average male life expectancy is around 75. You might just get there – this book will help.
- *5–9* Provided you're right about your family history and not a compulsive liar, it's looking good. Pass this book on to one of your pasty-looking friends.
- *1–4* Your lifestyle and genetic profile suggest a very long life – watch out for that bus!

What next? How long have you got – long enough to read this book? It's short and it's easy.

Top 20 health tips

In the time I've been writing about men's health I've come across a lot of good health advice and many useful tips. I've also come across a lot of rubbish, but you'd expect no less. The other day I saw a copy of a magazine promising an incredible 1,633 tips for better health – yes, 1,633! Hopeless – it's nowhere near as complicated as that.

I have a more realistic list of 20 tips for you to consider. (Actually, there are 21 – lucky this isn't a maths book.) You probably already know a lot of them, and others are included in the 'How long have I got?' checklist on pp. 1–2. Some of them are official Government policy, and some sound more like slogans or sayings. All of them are based on sound scientific evidence.

1 Eat five portions of fruit and veg a day.

2   Eat fish (but not deep fried in batter) at least twice a week.
3   Eat red meat no more than twice a week.
4   Don't drink more than three or four units of alcohol a day.
5   Don't binge drink.
6   Don't smoke.
7   Although the odd puff won't kill you, don't do drugs as a life-style choice.
8   Avoid addiction by knowing the difference between you controlling your behaviour and your behaviour controlling you.
9   Get some exercise every day.
10 Get at least three 20-minute aerobic exercise sessions a week.
11 Know the risks of unprotected sex.
12 Check out the risks of whatever you want to do before you do it (or, more simply, look before you leap).
13 If you're angry, try to think about it before acting on it – leave the room or count to ten.
14 Whether it's meditation or macramé, swimming or singing, find something that relaxes you and do it regularly.
15 Get a good night's sleep.
16 Don't overwork – regularly working more than 40 hours a week is bad for your health.
17 Read – it keeps the brain active, helps sleep and is a natural relaxant.
18 Get a bit of sun every day.
19 Walk – it's good for the heart and lungs and improves brain function by boosting its oxygen supply.
20 Make sure you know at least five people who you actually can – and do – talk to.
21 If you're ill, see your GP.

True, some of these are easier said than done, but all of them are more pleasant than three hours of chemotherapy – trust me on that.

How many of them do you do? But if you do all of them nearly all the time, you're probably not reading this book. If you don't do them because you can't see how to fit them into your life, you don't know why they will help or you simply can't be bothered, then read on. Chapter 3 will show you how to build all of them into your life, without changing who you are or what you do. It will also explain those that aren't obvious.

But give us the numbers – how much will doing all this healthy stuff really help?

This is the question every man wants answered and, until recently, it was difficult to give a good reply. In 2008, however, the results of a study that began in the early 1990s in Norfolk were published. The study followed 20,000 people over 45 for a decade. The researchers gave participants one point for:

- not currently smoking
- drinking fewer than 14 units of alcohol per week
- eating five servings of fruit and vegetables each day
- not being inactive (that is, taking just half an hour basic exercise a day).

The key number here is four. Those who did all four of the above were four times less likely to die during the ten year study than those who did none of them.

To be more specific, a 60-year-old person with a score of zero had the same risk of dying as a 74-year-old with all four points. So, the answer to the question is that doing all this healthy stuff will add about 14 years to your life. Fourteen years is a lot. You might even live to see one of the home nations win the World Cup. (OK, probably not that long, but you know what I'm saying.)

Another way of looking at it – as they did in a 40-year study of 6,000 Americans of Japanese origin published in 2006 – is that if in mid-life you're basically doing the healthy things, then you have a 60 per cent chance of survival to 85. If you have the full set of bad habits, then you have just a one in ten chance of reaching 85. Any gambler will tell you that there's a big difference between 6–4 on and 10–1.

Isn't it all in the genes?

Genes are a factor, but the Norfolk survey actually proves that changing lifestyle alone can add years to your life. If you're lucky with your genes too, well, who knows how long you could go on. Scientists reckon that there's no reason why the human body shouldn't last 120 years or so.

These are the factors that influence your health:

- the hand you're playing (including your genes, age and sex)
- your lifestyle
- the access you have to services
- your social and economic position
- your environment.

The first two are by far the most important. True, there's not a lot you can do to change the hand you've been dealt, but you can find out how good or bad a hand it is simply by checking your family history. Poker players know a bit about risk, and any half decent one will tell you that you need to know how good or bad your hand is before even considering whether you want to gamble on it.

Heart disease, cancer and stroke – the biggest killers – run in families (see 'Know the risks' box). So, often, do mental health problems like depression. Find out whether your parents, grand-parents, aunts and uncles have had any of these illnesses, especially if they died young. I had cancer in my thirties. My mum has had cancer and my grandmother died young from a different type of cancer. That simple level of detail is really all you need. Make sure that your GP knows your family health history.

Know the risks

Here are the five killers of men that you need to know about.

Heart disease
Heart disease is the main cause of male death. You have a 3–1 chance of dying from a heart or circulatory disease sooner or later. For too many men, it's sooner. A man dies prematurely from a heart-related disease every 14 minutes in the UK. Most heart attacks – at least 70 per cent – occur in men, but even this most obvious sign of heart disease needn't kill if you know what to do. (See box 'Am I having a heart attack?' on p. 90 in Chapter 4.)

Cancer
This is the other major killer. Take out the cancers that just affect women (like breast cancer) or men (like prostate cancer), and men are at greater risk than women. Among young people in England

and Wales (under 65s), 63 per cent more men get cancers that should be affecting men and women equally.

You have a 3–1 chance of getting cancer at some time in your life and a 4–1 chance of dying from it. Men die prematurely from cancer even more often than from heart disease – one death every 12.5 minutes. There is no need for this to be the case. Cancer is not the killer it once was; more than half of the people who get cancer are still alive five years later. Early diagnosis is everything.

Respiratory disease

You have a 5–1 chance of dying from a respiratory disease of the lungs and/or airways. The UK's death rate from respiratory disease is almost double the European average. The main cause of respiratory disease in you and those around you is smoking.

Accidents

Men are twice as likely to die in an accident as women, and they are three times more likely to die in a road accident. Is it really twice as dangerous to be a man in the modern world as a woman? No – it's just that a lot of men don't understand risk. Incredible as it may sound, unintentional injuries cause about half of the deaths in men under 25.

Suicide

Men are three times more likely to commit suicide than women. In England and Wales, a man takes his own life every three hours. Suicide rates are higher for men than women in most societies (China is a rare exception). Nine suicides in ten are the result of mental illness, notably depression.

By contrast, your lifestyle is pretty much entirely in your hands. I'm talking about things such as diet, exercise, smoking, drinking, drugs, sexual behaviour, your personality, your attitude to risk and your attitude to yourself and others. That's what this book is mainly about. To get an idea of the balance between lifestyle and family history, it is estimated that four out of five cancers can be prevented. In other words, 80 per cent of cancers are down to lifestyle, so there's a lot you can do.

There's no hard line between lifestyle and genes anyway – lifestyle factors are often the trigger to a genetic predisposition. In other words, lung cancer may be in your genes, but if you don't smoke you may well never trigger it.

When looking at the factors that affect your health, it is important also to bear in mind access to health services. Access for men has improved over the past few years. For example, most GP surgeries are now open outside working hours.

Knowing what to do when you have a problem can make all the difference – perhaps the difference between life and death. Do you know how many of the people who have heart attacks are still alive a month later? More than you might think – half of them. The key factor, as with all health problems, is early intervention. (See box 'Am I having a heart attack?' on p. 90 in Chapter 4.)

If sex influences health, then is the male naturally weaker than the female?

The answer to this is probably. Our genetic information – DNA – is carried in our cells in chromosomes. Women have two X chromosomes, which support each other; a flaw in one may be compensated for by the other. Because we have an X chromosome and a Y, we don't have this built-in support. In practice this means that eggs fertilized by sperm carrying a Y chromosome (potential boys) are more likely to self-abort. If they make it to term, then boys are more likely to die at birth.

Perhaps male weakness is the reason why, in most societies in most times, more boys are born than girls (about 105–107 boys to every 100 girls). In later life, having only one X chromosome may make men more vulnerable to genetic diseases such as heart disease.

Some scientists, such as Brian Sykes (a genetics professor at Oxford University), reckon that the Y chromosome is so flaky that eventually men will die out. Sykes gives us 125,000 years.

What's this about social and economic position?

Put bluntly, rich people tend to live longer than poor people. In the UK, women tend to live four to five years longer than men, but if you compare women on high incomes with men on low incomes the gap is nearer to 12 years. In fact, men on lower incomes have a shorter life expectancy in 2008 than the average woman had in

1952. Shockingly, there are parts of the UK where the life expectancy of a boy born today is less than 55 years.

But even this is more complicated than it appears. Although there is a link between wealth and health – the wealthier are healthier – there is an even stronger link between happiness and health. In other words, happy people are more likely to be healthy than wealthy people. Of course, it's not easy to be happy when you've got no job or a job you don't like, but it does prove that simply focusing on getting a better job is not the way to go. There's more to think about than this, as you'll see in the rest of this book.

So should you risk reading on? The next section will help you to decide.

Why you should risk reading on

- Cancer: 3–1
- Winning the lottery: 14,000,000–1

This is a short book about men's health. I've already listed the basic health tips that will maximize your chances of good health and a long life (see 'Top 20 health tips', on p. 3). So you could stop reading now if you wanted to, but if you do you won't find out why most men don't do these things and, most importantly, how you can do them yourself without changing your lifestyle.

You've probably heard some of the health tips before. You're probably a bit sceptical about some of them. Perhaps you think it's all a bit more complicated than that; we're all individuals – it's not the same for everyone. To some extent you'd be right. Oversimplification of health messages doesn't help anyone, and at times health campaigners have been guilty of this. But that's not a problem – this book will explain any little complexities and enable you to make your own decisions.

The truth is that it's not scepticism about the messages that prevents us from acting on them. It's more that we can't be bothered. We don't think it will happen to us. Be honest, can you really imagine the world without you? I can't. Most of us can't. So we risk it.

Risk is a part of life and, for whatever reason, it's usually a bigger part of a man's life than a woman's. We take risks because of hormones, especially testosterone. We take risks because of the adrenaline rush. We take risks because society expects it (boys will be boys), and we take risks because it's fun. We shouldn't feel bad about this – being male isn't an illness after all – but we do need to understand it.

Sometimes, all of these risk-taking impulses combine to make us do some very daft and dangerous things. For some men it appears that unless they've actually seen the blood-splattered carnage of a road accident at 70 mph, they can't conceive of just how ugly it might be. This lack of imagination has served men – and women – well over millions of years. It is very useful before fighting a sabre-tooth tiger, for example, or riding off into the sunset to seek out new worlds and new civilizations, or charging into battle in a war. But what are the risks you need to run in the modern world? Not so many. That's why spectator sports are so popular – we identify with one team or performer and get our risk-taking thrills second hand. (Men experience a testosterone surge when their team wins, just as they would if they won themselves.)

It's also why we like to try 'extreme' sports. Do you think that a man just back from a war would care about kite-surfing? Of course not. These things are substitutes, and there are many more that are easier (and cheaper) than kite-surfing: binge drinking, drug taking, shagging like a demented rabbit and so on. I'm not saying that there's anything necessarily wrong with these or any other risks you might want to take, but I am saying that you should understand what they're all about – your biological urge to take risk.

Risk-taking is normal in adolescence. When you're a teenager you have a sudden rush of hormones pushing you in all directions. At the same time, the parts of the brain that deal with judgement and impulse control haven't yet fully developed. When they do develop, most people grow out of these behaviours. This is also why you need to be careful about what you get into as a teenager. Start to smoke and you'll be a nicotine addict within a year, probably a lot quicker. Start drinking seriously at 14 and your risk of becoming addicted to alcohol is four times greater than if you start at 20. In other words, experimenting as a teenager is fine, but if you adopt a lifestyle at this age it can be very difficult to shake off.

Some social scientists have argued that because kids today get to take fewer risks than children of previous generations, they're less able to make judgements as adults. I don't know whether that's true but I do know that excessive risk-taking is killing men before their time.

As I've already said, every year in the UK about 120,000 men die prematurely. This death toll is totally unnecessary – men are not biologically programmed to keel over at the age of 75. There is no good reason why we shouldn't live as long as women do, but we don't. The world has changed but we have not changed with it.

We need to get smart. Run risks that are worth running for the right reasons. Find out the facts, make your own choices and be prepared to change your mind when more information comes along. These are far more useful skills, ones that will be valued more highly by men and women alike. Nobody is saying that you shouldn't jump out of a plane – just think about it for long enough to make sure that you've got your parachute on and know how to use it. When it comes to the risks you run with your health, this book is that parachute!

When even the editor of that most laddish of lad mags *Loaded* says, as Martin Daubney did in 2005, that 'men have realized that if they adopt the ways of the gays, they get laid more often', perhaps the writing is on the wall for full-on laddishness. 'It is Darwinian evolution,' says Daubney. So evolve, guys!

2

The key applications inside out

The brain

You're nothing without the stuff between your ears. Your heart can sometimes be kick-started back into life, but once your brain's gone so are you.

Specifications

- *Weight of adult brain*: 1.4 kg.
- *Material*: not grey or white matter but a soft red jelly protected by a hard bone case (skull).
- *Structure*: there are five main parts. The *cerebellum* and *brain stem* control the basic functions we're unaware of, such as breathing and balance. At the core of the brain, these haven't evolved much and are pretty similar in all mammals. The evolved part that does the thinking stuff is called the *cerebrum*. The cerebrum makes up about three-quarters of the brain's weight. The other two parts are the *hypothalamus*, which controls temperature, and the *pituitary gland*, a pea-sized blob in the middle of the brain that controls your hormones.
- *Number of cells*: 100 billion nerve cells (neurones) plus several hundred billion support cells. Each cell connects to about 25,000 others.

System requirements

- *Good, oxygenated blood.* The brain takes about 20 per cent of the heart's blood output. Strokes – the third major killer of men – occur when arteries are blocked and blood can't reach the brain. Strokes affect men of all ages.

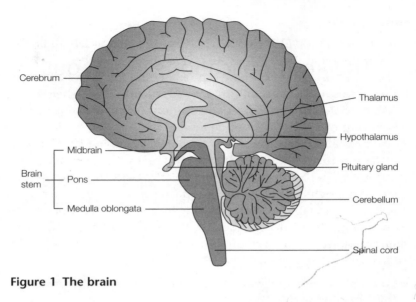

Figure 1 The brain

- *Protection*. Because the brain is both very complicated and cased in a hard shell, repairing it is very difficult indeed. So protecting it from getting damaged in the first place by wearing a helmet, for example, when biking or boarding is essential. Concussion can be dangerous. If you're knocked out even for a moment, see a doctor, and make sure that you recover fully. A second injury while recovering from a first may be more permanent.
- *Exercise*. Like all muscles in your body, use it or lose it. Crosswords, poker, learning languages, reading Proust, trying to understand how the Large Hadron Collider works, trying to understand how your TV remote control works – it's your choice, but whatever you do make sure you use your brain.
- *Good quality neurotransmitters*. Neurotransmitters are the chemicals the brain needs to function well. They carry signals between brain cells. Like all chemicals in the body, they can only be formed from the ingredients you make available – in other words, from what you eat.

How it works

The cerebrum is divided into two halves – the famous left and right sides of the brain. Each side is subdivided into four lobes.

The most important of these is probably the frontal lobe. It does the concentrating, plans and makes judgements. This where most of what's different between us and chimps – with whom we share 99 per cent of our DNA – is to be found.

We hear a lot about the two sides of the brain, but it's complex and, despite the application of many great brains to the problem, we still don't know exactly how our brain works. Generally, the left side controls the right side of the body and *vice versa*. In addition, everyone has a dominant half – the left side in the 90 per cent of people who are right-handed – that deals with speech, writing, maths and the sensible stuff, whereas the other side is more artistic, creative and generally concerned with colours, sounds and shapes.

High-performance brain

The brain has a processing power about 100,000 times faster than the best computer. But because we're constantly multitasking – one-third of the brain is taken up simply with processing what we see, for example – the difference in outputs is less obvious. Neurones communicate with each other using electrically powered chemicals called neurotransmitters. Neurones can fire neurotransmitters several times a second at speeds of up to 267 mph.

Frequently asked questions

Is it true that we only use ten per cent of our brain?

No. We only use about ten per cent of our neurones at any one time, but most of the brain sees action at some point during the day or night.

Do we lose millions of brain cells each day?

This is a bit of a myth too. Brain cells don't die as we age, they just shrivel. As a result, the brain does get a little smaller over the years but the neurones stick around, provided you don't have a specific disease that kills them. Smoking and alcohol have also been shown to destroy brain cells.

Are men's brains bigger than women's?

Yes, about nine per cent bigger – but don't draw any conclusions from this about intelligence. Einstein's brain was about 14 per cent smaller than average (1230 g compared with 1400 g), whereas the bottle-nosed dolphin's brain is slightly larger than the average human's. Neanderthal man probably had larger brains than us too.

Men's brains are different from women's as a result of the testosterone that kicks in during the second trimester of pregnancy, but your brain started out exactly the same as a girl's – female is the default setting for brains and, indeed, pretty much everything else. All of us were girls before we became boys.

What can go wrong with the brain?

Brain tumours are up (by 45 per cent in the past 30 years). So is Alzheimer's disease, affecting two to five per cent of people over 65. We don't know much about what causes either. Why? Because frankly we don't really know much about how the brain works. It's for this reason that you need to think seriously before taking drugs like cannabis, LSD, ketamine and others. The long-term – and sometimes even the short-term – effects are highly unpredictable.

However, by far the single biggest preventable problem concerns our mental health. At least one in six and perhaps as many as one in four of us have depression or other mental health problems at some time in our lives. (There's more on this in the section 'Depression: as dangerous as smoking?' on p. 77.)

How do you tell the difference between dementia and a bad memory?

It's not easy. My grandad had a brilliant memory but dementia in later life. For a while, his memory for things he was interested in – odds on horses, for example – disguised the deeper problem.

Absent-mindedness is normal when you're busy. Forgetting names is normal. More worrying is forgetting where you are – especially getting lost in familiar surroundings – or forgetting to put on clothes before going out.

Forgetting where you put things is normal – putting them in a totally inappropriate place (like flowers in the fridge) is more worrying. Forgetting a word happens to us all; doing it habitually and substituting other less suitable ones is more worrying.

Even the smartest people can get dementia. Fantasy writer Terry Pratchett has an imagination most of us can only wonder at, but he was diagnosed with a form of Alzheimer's disease at the age of 59. Early onset dementia like this is very rare, but if you're concerned then get advice sooner rather than later.

How do I improve my memory?

Keep your mind active by using it (see system requirements above). Here are five ways to develop a better memory.

1 Reproducing information helps it stick. Use more than one sense. If someone tells you something, write it down. If you're reading something, say it out loud. Take a mental picture of your keys on the table, or of information written down.
2 Don't rely on lists and diaries – read, visualize and leave them at home.
3 Group items. It's easier to remember three groups of three than one of nine. Alternatively, invent schoolboy rhymes. For example, 'while she's relaxing with a bit of Fay Weldon, check out your symptoms in Jim's book from Sheldon.'
4 Say things you need to remember aloud to yourself or someone else.
5 Er, there is another one. It's really good. No – it's gone.

Is Mozart good for the brain?

Possibly. It appears that loudness cycles of 20–30 seconds mirror the brain's natural rhythms, so it's probably the variations in volume – more common in classical music than pop – rather than the music itself that helps.

The heart

A fist-sized bag of pumping muscle protected by your rib cage, the heart is the body's most important organ. Its job is nothing more

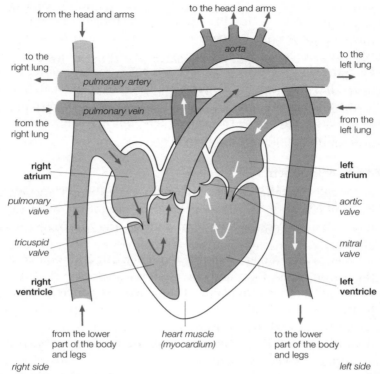

Figure 2 The heart

and nothing less than to keep you alive by pumping blood filled with oxygen around your body. It does this around 60–90 times a minute, depending on how old you are, how fit you are and what you're doing.

It may only be the size of a fist, but a healthy heart punches well above its weight. It's good for more beats than a DJs' convention – pumping billions and billions of times during the course of a lifetime. What's your BPM (beats per minute)? You can find out by taking your pulse.

Specifications

- *Weight of an adult heart*: 300 g.
- *Material*: mainly a special type of muscle called myocardium.
- *Size*: approximately 13 cm high by 9 cm wide and 6 cm deep.

- *Structure*: a double-action in/out pump with four separate chambers.
- *BPM at rest*: 60–90.
- *Amount of blood pumped per minute at rest*: about 6 litres (nearly 13 pints).
- *BPM when exercising*: up to 200 or more.
- *Amount of blood pumped per minute when exercising*: 50 litres (106 pints) or more.
- *Beats in the average lifetime*: 25,000,000,000.

System requirements

- *Fresh air.* Cigarette smoke, pollution, car exhausts and other harmful chemicals in the air make it harder for the heart to do its job. They all cause long-term damage and can trigger heart attacks.
- *A balanced diet.* A diet including too much salt and too many of the wrong types of fats and cholesterols can clog up the arteries with a substance called plaque. Plaque sets like concrete, making it harder for the heart to do its job. Again, this can cause long-term damage and trigger heart attacks.
- *A healthy weight.* The heavier you are, the harder your heart has to work to move you about.
- *Regular exercise.* To beat at its best over a whole lifetime, the heart needs to work out regularly at different rates, including resting, walking, running and exercising. Men in active occupations have half the risk of heart disease of those in inactive ones. So, if you have a sitting down job you need to get up and get moving to make up for it. There's more about safe exercising on p. 52 ('Exercise: want to get back in the game?').
- *A relaxed attitude.* Stress will increase blood pressure. Blood pressure will increase your risk of heart problems, so relax. Nothing's worth having a heart attack for. It's not the end of the world (unless it is the end of the world, in which case it doesn't matter).

How it works

The heart is such a masterpiece of engineering that it makes the engine of a Ferrari look like a broken hair-dryer.

There are two pumps. One pump (on the left side of the heart) sends blood full of oxygen down the arteries into the body. Once it has distributed its oxygen, the blood comes back to the heart down the veins. The other pump (on the right) redirects this blood to the lungs, where it picks up more oxygen and the whole process starts again.

But what keeps it going?

Electricity. The heart has its own tiny pacemaker on the top of the right side of the heart that produces a series of tiny electrical pulses. It's these that you feel when you take your 'pulse' and these that you see as waves on an electrocardiogram scan. You've probably seen TV doctors shouting 'clear!' and trying to restart a heart by passing a massive electrical current through it. It's this pacemaker that they're trying to spark back into action.

So why is the heart such a funny shape – why isn't it heart-shaped?

That's the really clever bit. The heart works without you really noticing it because the amount of blood pumped by one side exactly matches the amount pumped by the other. To do this the left side, which has to pump blood through the whole body, must work harder than the right side, which only has to pump blood into the lungs. As a result, the left side is more muscular and therefore bigger.

High-performance heart

The heart will pump 10,000 times or more without missing a beat, speeding up automatically when you need more oxygen for exercise and slowing down when you need less while sleeping. In return, all it needs from you is oxygen, water and a handful of nutrients (available from fruit and vegetables) three or four times a day – a lot cheaper than a gallon of petrol and usually tastier.

When exercised regularly the heart becomes larger, which means that each beat pumps more blood and thus more oxygen around the body.

Giving up smoking will see your risk of heart disease reduced to that of a non-smoker within three to five years, which is proof of the heart's strength and resilience.

Frequently asked questions

Why do men get heart disease?

Men are at more risk from heart disease because the female hormone oestrogen protects women. Heart disease will kill at least a third of men, and the rate in the UK is higher than the rate in other countries in Europe.

The problem is that the arteries that carry blood from the heart are only as wide as a drinking straw and can easily become blocked up with plaque – a substance containing calcium and cholesterol, which sets like concrete. Plaque increases with age, so the less you produce when you're younger the better.

Weight is also important, especially in men. Whereas women get fat around the hips and bum, men get fat around the middle, closer to the internal organs like the heart and therefore more likely to damage them. Blood is also more likely to clot in obese people.

What's high blood pressure?

Blood pressure gives an insight into how hard the heart is working. It shoots up when you first wake and get up, for example. High pressure means it's being forced to work harder, which can increase the risk of heart problems.

Blood pressure is shown as two figures. The first refers to when the heart is tightening and the second to when it is relaxing. For a healthy young male, 110/75 is normal (you'll hear nurses, doctors and actors on *ER* say 'bp – 110 over 75'). For a man of 60, it may be nearer 150/90.

High blood pressure is often hereditary, so make sure that your GP knows if people in your family tend to have high blood pressure. If you're not sure, have a look at your fingerprints. The more swirly they are, the more likely you are to have high blood pressure.

The penis and testicles

The penis, as you've probably discovered, is used for peeing, making babies and generally having fun with. You're very lucky to have one, so take care of it.

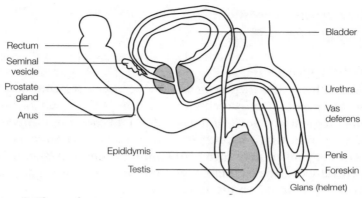

Figure 3 The male sex organs

You get an erection when the small muscles in your penis, which are usually tightly contracted, relax and allow blood to flow in. The spongy tissue in the penis fills with blood and expands, pushing against the veins and closing them so the blood cannot drain out again – all very romantic.

As editor of <malehealth.co.uk>, I get more questions about male apparatus than any other subject. I'll try to answer as many of them as possible here.

Specifications

- *Size*: most penises, when they're erect, are about the same length (between about five and a half and six and a quarter inches long). However, the exact size varies a lot, according to who measures it. In surveys when a doctor measures, penis size drops by up to 50 per cent compared with surveys in which the owner measures it.
- *Material*: the penis is composed of three cylinders of spongy erectile tissue full of blood vessels.
- *Structure*: the urethra, the body's outlet tube for both sperm and urine (although only one at a time), passes through the middle of the smallest of these cylinders – the corpus spongiosum – which is found on the underside of the penis. The corpus spongiosum expands at the tip to form the head of the penis, called the glans. The glans is protected by the foreskin.

- *Output*: each ejaculation of semen contains about 200–300 million sperm.
- *Performance*: variable.

System requirements

- All of the system requirements for the heart (see above) apply to the penis. Why? Because an erection is the result of blood flooding into the penis. If the blood is not flowing properly, then the erection won't happen properly. The blood pressure inside an erect penis is very high – 700 mmHg or more (140 mmHg is generally considered 'high' blood pressure). It takes a good, efficiently pumping heart to provide this.
- *Temperature*. Some like it hot but not sperm. They thrive at about three degrees below body temperature. This is why your testicles, which house your sperm factory, are outside the body. It also means baggy trousers and boxers are best for baby making.

Routine maintenance

- Keep your penis clean, including under the foreskin. It is naturally smelly at best, and after a day or so that nasty white stuff – smegma – starts to bloom. This can lead to a swollen glans (helmet), or balanitis (literally, 'inflammation of the acorn'). Frequent washing with plain soap and a couple of handfuls of salt in the bath should sort it out. If not, see your GP. Balanitis may also be caused by perfumes in soaps and gels or sex with a woman who has thrush. Poor hygiene can also increase the risk of cancer of the penis, although this is very rare.
- Look after the groin area too. 'Jock itch', which is caused by the same tinea fungus as athlete's foot, thrives in warm, moist conditions – a good description of the average man's pants. Wash with unperfumed soaps, dry thoroughly and – superheroes take note – avoid tight nylon underpants. See your GP if the problem persists.
- If you're not trying to have a baby, wear a condom to protect against STDs (sexually transmitted diseases) and HIV.

How it works

Sperm are manufactured in the testicles and pass along the epididymis, where mature sperm hang out. The epididymis is a microscopically narrow tube that is 6 m long, folded into a space of 5 cm – an engineering masterpiece.

Just before orgasm, the sperm travel along two narrow tubes of muscle called the vas deferens. These meet with the seminal vesicles, which are behind the bladder and just above the prostate gland. The seminal vesicles and the prostate gland add their own secretions to the semen. These fluids are alkaline, which protect the sperm from the acid in the vagina. At orgasm, the semen is propelled from two ejaculatory ducts along the urethra, which runs the length of the penis, and out of the urethral opening.

High performance penis and testicles

The average ejaculation contains 200–300 million sperm, but it only takes one to fertilize the egg. (This is just as well because only about 40 of them will get anywhere near the end of the race.)

Sperm are tadpole-shaped and about 0.05 mm long. From puberty onward, at least 1,000 sperm are manufactured each minute in the testicles. They take about two and a half months to mature and spend the last couple of weeks in the epididymis.

Sperm swim at about 15 cm a second but at the point of ejaculation they are propelled a lot faster – about 28 mph – along with the rest of the seminal fluid. Two minutes after entering the female, they're at the cervix and five minutes later at the fallopian tubes.

During the most fertile part of the female menstrual cycle (period), this journey is much easier because at this time there is plenty of fertile mucus around for the sperm to live off. They can survive like this for – take a deep breath, non-condom users – a week. The woman's most fertile period is when the egg is released – usually between the 12th and 18th day of the cycle. If you and your partner are trying for a baby, this is when you'll be at it like Olympic athletes.

Frequently asked questions

Is my penis too small?

Penises come in all shapes and sizes, with bumps and bends and visible veins – the lot. Genuine problems that might actually stop you peeing or enjoying sex are rare and usually picked up when you're very young, so if you got through the nappy stage then you're probably good to go.

If you're worried about your penis size, have a proper look at it. When you look at your penis normally, you're looking down on it. It's like looking down on someone from the top of a building. Even basketball players look small when you look down on them from above.

Hold a mirror at the side and have a proper look. That's more the sort of view you get of another man's penis in the public lavatory. Honestly, very, very few men are over- or under-endowed to the point that they cannot enjoy great sex. Think about it – the vagina can be big enough to let a baby out or small enough to hold a tampon, which means it can cope with any size without loss of performance.

Operations to enlarge the penis tend only to make it look bigger when limp and not when erect, and are – like any other surgery – potentially dangerous. You only have one penis. Although livers, kidneys and hearts can all be replaced if necessary through transplants, the penis cannot.

Why is my erect penis bent?

Every penis is a bit bent, and a slight bend upward is not just normal but desirable. However, if your penis is bent to the left or right so much that it is difficult or even painful to enter your partner during sex, this could be a condition called Peyronie's disease (not an Italian beer). If the 'bend' is severe, surgery can improve matters. Men aged 50 to 60 are most at risk, although Peyronie's can occur in men of all ages.

Why can't I get an erection?

Not getting an erection when you want one is usually called ED (erectile dysfunction). Impotence is a popular word for this problem but not the right one because the problem can nearly always be solved.

The official estimate is that ED affects about one in ten men at any one time. (The incidence increases from about one in 13 in men under 30 to one in two in men over 70.) Some surveys, however, have put it as high as one in four. Either way, nearly all men suffer from ED from time to time.

ED is one of the things about being a flesh and blood human rather than a robot. Men who expect their penises to work like machines have not learned that yet. Don't worry about it but don't ignore it either. If it keeps happening, see a doctor. Why? Because ED can be an early warning of some serious health problems including:

- heart disease;
- narrow arteries;
- high blood pressure;
- diabetes;
- Peyronie's disease;
- multiple sclerosis;
- an injury to the pelvis or spinal cord;
- heavy drinking or smoking; or
- drugs – either the side effects of prescribed drugs (e.g. some anti-depressants and drugs for hypertension) or the abuse of non-prescribed drugs.

Low testosterone levels are seldom the cause of ED. Although a low testosterone level may reduce your desire to go out and seek sex, it won't affect erections when sex is in front of you. In other words, even if you have low testosterone levels, seeing something you find sexually exciting should prompt an erection.

Research suggests that men don't seek help with ED because they don't think it can be treated. This is not true – there are many causes of ED, physical and psychological, but it can nearly always be treated. There is usually some physical cause for ED; it is purely psychological in only about 25 per cent of cases. Whatever the cause, worrying about sexual performance can make it worse. This is because anxiety contracts the muscles, preventing blood from entering the penis.

If you get erections at night or when masturbating but have problems with your partner, it's almost certainly not a physical problem so just relax. The chances are you'll live to at least 80, so there's plenty of time.

As usual, smoking is a no-no. Nicotine interferes with the flow of blood to the penis, making an erection less likely. Smokers are

50–80 per cent more likely to have ED than non-smokers. Engrave it on your lighter.

ED can be treated using drugs that your doctor can prescribe. You may be tempted to buy these off the internet, but you should only do this if you already have a doctor's prescription. Sites that will sell you drugs without a prescription could, frankly, be selling you anything, including fakes made with blue paint and pesticides. Also, if you don't see a doctor, the underlying causes – which may be far more serious than a bit of brewer's droop – won't be sorted out.

There's an excellent section on <malehealth.co.uk> about ED drugs, including what Viagra, Cialis and the various other types do, as well as information on safe online buying.

If you have the opposite problem, an erection all the time, this could be priapism – a painful condition that requires prompt treatment to avoid the risk of ED in the future and permanent damage to the penis. As a guide, any man whose erection continues for four hours or more should see a doctor.

If testosterone has nothing to do with erections, what is it for?

Testosterone is the most important of the male hormones. It's made mostly in the testicles but also in the adrenal glands. (The ovaries and adrenal glands produce it in lower levels in women.) In men, it is responsible for muscle, bone and sexual development, as well as sex drive. At puberty, it makes the voice drop and the penis, testicles, and facial and pubic hair grow.

Women's hormones have been at the forefront of health for decades now. Only recently have the hormonal fluctuations that men experience attracted any interest. But the fact is that male mood, behaviour and, indeed, health are heavily influenced by our hormones, especially testosterone. Testosterone levels fluctuate according to circumstances. They can rise before and, if successful, after conflict. They can fall after marriage or the birth of a child.

Overall testosterone levels fall slightly with age. Some men – particularly those with high levels to begin with – can effectively have half as much testosterone in their blood at 80 as at 20. It may lead to loss of muscle tone and bone strength, and increased weight and risk of heart disease and diabetes.

Whether reduced testosterone is the cause of the sluggishness, loss of libido and depression that some middle-aged men experience or is the result of it is debatable. (Depressed men often have low levels of testosterone and high levels of cortisol, which is the hormone released in response to stress.) Testosterone replacement therapy is available but, while trials continue, many doctors are sceptical.

Can you boost testosterone levels naturally?

Yes. By taking more exercise, having more sex, making sure you get your essential fatty acids (see section 'Eating: want weight loss without great loss?' on p. 37) and getting a good night's sleep (see box 'Zzzzz: tips for getting some shut-eye' on p. 112). Also, fat reduces the amount of testosterone available to the body, so losing weight and cutting down on fatty foods and beer may help.

Eat more seeds (particularly pumpkin and sunflower seeds), shellfish, beans, yoghurt and lean meat. These are high in zinc, which is the mineral that is essential for testosterone production. Broccoli, cauliflower, radishes, turnips, cabbage and Brussels sprouts can help too, as can ginseng, the South American herb Muira Puama and even stinging nettles (safer in a tea than raw).

Are sperm counts falling?

They appear to be. Research suggests that during the past 50 years or so, the number of sperm in the average Western male's semen has halved. What doctors call a 'normal' sperm level today is just a third of the 'normal' level in the 1940s.

These days, the man will be the cause of the problem in around half of infertility cases, with about 70 per cent of male infertility problems being caused by low sperm count. All of the following can reduce sperm count:

- anabolic steroids (very severely);
- anti-arthritis drugs;
- alcohol;
- cocaine;
- chemotherapy;
- frequent marijuana use;

- low levels of minerals such as zinc;
- low levels of vitamins, particularly vitamin C;
- smoking (reduces the sperm's life expectancy and sense of direction);
- some other prescription drugs (this includes, according to recent research, ED drugs like Viagra, which is a good argument against 'recreational' use of these drugs by men who might want to start families);
- stress; and
- a vasectomy, which may not be as reversible as is sometimes believed.

It's not clear whether falling sperm counts are linked to the increase in testicular cancer. Although still rare, it has more than doubled in the same time that sperm counts have halved.

Should I check my testicles for cancer?

The best way to monitor your own body for ill health is simply to be aware of it. Testicular cancer is rare and, if caught in time, nearly always treatable. Because of this, although it's still the main cancer among young men, more men die of breast cancer than testicular cancer. Rather than checking your testicles religiously and fretting over whether you're doing it properly, just be aware. Watch out for lumps or heaviness, and if you're concerned see your GP.

The prostate

The prostate – is that a sex organ?

We don't actually know its exact function but it certainly plays a big part in sex. The prostate is one organ where size does matter, and in this case small is beautiful.

It sits between the bladder and urethra (the tube through which you pee) and provides some of the fluids that make up the semen when you ejaculate. It contracts during orgasm, probably heightening the pleasure.

About the size of a walnut in an adult, it can grow to the size of a lemon or orange. This growth can make peeing difficult, reduce your interest in sex and cause erection problems.

What makes it grow?

The growth is related to testosterone. In the prostate gland, testosterone is broken down into the related hormone dihydro-testosterone, which appears to be involved in both baldness and the enlarged prostate. This doesn't mean that high or low levels of testosterone cause prostate cancer – or baldness, for that matter. It's more about the way your body reacts to a normal amount.

Most prostates grow. Although the growth is not caused by cancer, in some cases it can become cancerous. Very small cancers are sometimes seen even in young men after they die (from something else). By the age of 70, two men in three will have some degree of prostate cancer. The question is whether your prostate cancer is aggressive enough to kill you before something else does.

Doctors will often follow a treatment they like to call 'watchful waiting', which basically means doing nothing but carrying out regular tests. It's very common in prostate growth. They're trying to work out whether the growth has become cancerous and how quickly the cells are multiplying. Generally, the younger you are, the more aggressive a cancer is likely to be. Recent research has also suggested taller men might be more likely to have more aggressive cancers.

There's a strong family link. Your risk of prostate cancer is doubled if you have an affected brother or father, and it increases still further with the number of male relatives you have with the disease.

How dangerous is it?

After lung cancer, prostate cancer is the most common cancer killer of men in the UK, killing over 10,000 a year. It is still rare in men under 50.

Signs of a prostate problem include:

- a weak flow;
- intermittency – a flow which stops and starts;
- hesitancy – having to wait before you start to go;
- frequency – having to urinate more often than previously;
- urgency – finding it difficult to postpone urination; and
- nocturia – having to get up at night to urinate.

If you have these symptoms and want to know whether they're likely to be prostate related, ask yourself another question; is it easier and more satisfying peeing after having an orgasm? Some people with prostate problems find that it is, presumably as a result of the gland shrinking a little after it has added its vital fluid to your ejaculation.

What is good for the prostate?

We're not sure. There is a lot of research, with sometimes contradictory results, into what could be a 'prostate-friendly' diet. After reading a lot of it, I called the man who should know. As statistical epidemiologist at Cancer Research UK's unit at Oxford University, Andrew Roddam keeps an eye on all of these studies. What is his recommended prostate-friendly diet? The ordinary healthy diet that you all know about – or can read about in the section 'Eating: want weight loss without great loss?' (see p. 37) – without an excess of anything.

The big problem in prostate cancer research, more than in any other field, is that research tends to look at older men, but the key period that makes a difference could well come earlier in life, even in childhood.

However, one thing that does appear to help the prostate in the long term is frequent ejaculation through sex or masturbation when young. In an Australian study published in 2003, men who had ejaculated more than five times per week in their 20s were one-third less likely to develop aggressive prostate cancer later. So the prostate *is* a sex organ.

Networking with other systems: the ins and outs of sex

Regular sex is good for you, provided it's safe. It reduces stress, boosts the immune system, enhances self-esteem, aids sleep, burns calories and improves intimacy with your partner. It can even reduce pain. The way to make it 100 per cent safe is to use a condom.

I probably should have included the brain in this section on sex because that's the most important sex organ of all. Good sex happens in the head. I mean this in two ways – not just because so much of our sex lives involves fantasy, but also because good sex comes from feeling comfortable in ourselves about our bodies and our sexuality.

Celebrate your sexuality. 'Safe sex doesn't mean no sex, it just means use your imagination' is how Billy Bragg put it in his hit single 'Sexuality'. Like the bard of Barking says, your sexuality is all yours. It's part of you. Don't be ashamed of what you like.

The mouth is an important sex organ too – being able to talk honestly about sex with your partner is as important as doing it. Tell each other what you like. Do what you like, so long as it's legal and between consenting adults.

In the following sections I touch upon some issues that may not at first glance appear to have anything to do with your health (the subject of this book). However, I mention them because although they don't apply to everyone, they *can* have major implications for your mental and physical health.

Is masturbation bad for you?

No. It won't make you go blind, vote Monster Raving Looney or put you off your cornflakes. Most men masturbate and, despite what they might say, so do many women. It's perfectly normal. After all, our genitals are part of our bodies and pretty important to our future relationships, so it would be surprising if we weren't just a little curious about them.

In fact, masturbation can be good for you. It will help you to understand your body and your sexuality and what turns you on better. This may help you communicate with your partner more easily, enjoy sex more and avoid sex-related psychological problems. (Indeed, masturbating with your partner is a good way to show each other what you like.) Frequent orgasms also help to reduce the risk of prostate cancer, and masturbation itself also reduces the likelihood of phimosis – a tightness of the foreskin. Furthermore, although nobody has yet begun to promote masturbation as part of a calorie-controlled diet, David Haslam of the National Obesity Forum quotes a colleague who claims that five minutes of vigorous masturbation can consume 300 calories – the equivalent of sprinting 100 metres. The need for sexual pleasure is a natural human need, the same as the need for food and drink, and when the urge strikes it is better to masturbate than exploit someone else.

Having said all that, your penis is a delicate body part. Take care of it – don't stick it in anything other than your partner or stick anything else into it.

Anything that is enjoyable can become an addiction, and masturbation is no different. If it begins to interfere with the rest of your life and you're becoming more interested in it than in real sexual relationships with real people, then you need to be careful. If you can't stop, you need to. Just as for other addictions, there are organizations for people who are addicted in this way, such as Sexaholics Anonymous.

Is it OK to use pornography?

When you're a teenager, looking at porn is part of a normal curiosity, but using it when you're older depends more on your view of the politics of porn and its effect on society.

It is true that some women enjoy pornography aimed at heterosexual men, even including some of the women who appear, but – as with prostitution – this is the exception rather than the rule and there is a lot of abuse of women in the porn industry. Moreover, pornography, by definition, exploits women by treating them as objects for sexual pleasure. Because you can't avoid that, regular use may affect your attitudes to women and spoil your relationships with them.

Be careful – you can get addicted to pornography too. Read the interview with Jason on p. 74 (section entitled 'Addiction: how can something that felt so good feel so bad?').

What about prostitution?

At the time of writing, paying for sex is not illegal although selling it can be. The Government is considering changing the law. The difficulty is that the law on prostitution doesn't reflect the idea behind other sex laws, which is to protect people from being abused. Although some prostitutes may enjoy their work, many are abused or do it unwillingly.

What if what I like doing is illegal?

Then it gets more difficult. Historically, the law in most countries has been uncomfortable and confused about sexuality. This continues to this day, and in the UK both the Sexual Offences Act of 2003 and the Criminal Justice and Immigration Act of 2008 (which introduced a new offence of possession of extreme pornographic images) have been criticized for these reasons.

The law tries to look at the actors rather than the act. It tries to ensure that people are not abused. There are few acts between consenting adults that are illegal, but all this changes if the people involved are relatives or if one of them is under the age of consent (16 in the UK). It can be a confusing area but to put it bluntly in terms we all understand – if you're an adult and have sex with a child you're breaking the law.

Even if you want to have illegal sex such as sex with children, your sexuality – what you want to do – is not your fault. You didn't choose it. But you do have a legal responsibility not to act on your desires. You can get help. Difficult though it may be, you must try to do this before you commit illegal sex acts. Once you have abused a child, it becomes more difficult because you will also be treated as a criminal.

The Lucy Faithfull Foundation run a project called Stop it Now (<www.stopitnow.org.uk>), which has a helpline for people seeking help with stopping their own abusive behaviour (freephone 0808 1000 900). It also provides support for those who suspect someone they know presents a risk to children.

It's important to understand the difference between fantasy and reality in sexuality. You can fantasize about whatever you want. What may be illegal is acting it out. Pornography may help with your fantasy, but if in creating the images someone has been abused in reality, then a crime has been committed, and you're aiding and abetting that crime by using the image.

What are the symptoms of VD or a sexually transmitted disease?

STIs (sexually transmitted infections), formerly known as VD (venereal disease), are very common and can affect you whether you're straight, gay or bisexual. You don't need to have sex with lots of people to be at risk – just one brief encounter with a person with an STI may be enough.

There are several common STIs including herpes, genital warts, gonorrhoea ('the clap') and syphilis. HIV (the virus that causes AIDS) can also be transmitted through sex. Infections with chlamydia, the most common STI, are up 150 per cent since 1998.

As a rule, STIs can be safely treated if they're caught early. If not, they can become more serious, possibly causing infertility or even death.

STIs can be transmitted through vaginal sex, oral sex, anal sex and, in some cases, through skin-to-skin contact. (Note that HIV cannot be passed via skin-to-skin contact.)

Some of the more common symptoms to look out for include:

- a yellow discharge from your penis;
- swollen testicles;
- rashes or soreness in the penis or tackle region; and
- pain when peeing. (A short-term stinging sensation when peeing may be cystitis – drink plenty of water and it should improve.)

If you have any of these symptoms, or any other sexual health concerns, get them checked by a GP or a specialist genito-urinary medicine (GUM) clinic (see question 'Talking of sex, what about sexually transmitted infections?' on p. 93). You can buy self-testing kits in pharmacists, but use them with care. If you have one STI, you've quite possibly got another, so it still makes sense to see a doctor.

Don't buy STI treatments online. Research from 2007 found high prices and a lack of information about the products and their side effects. If you really need to do all this over the internet, try <drthom .com>. Their doctors are registered with the Healthcare Commission to provide sexual health testing and treatment by post.

The best way to avoid STIs is through safe sex. If you aren't safe and are concerned that you might have caught something, get yourself checked out, even if you don't have any symptoms. Some STIs such as chlamydia and even HIV often cause no symptoms at first.

Is blood at orgasm a symptom of an STI?

Blood in the semen can be very scary but is usually harmless. A bit of rough sex or masturbation may be the cause, although only one in five cases has an obvious cause. Very rarely it can be a sign of something more serious, so see a doctor if it keeps on happening.

What about blood when you pee?

Is it definitely blood? If you have not been drinking enough water your urine can begin to look brown. Certain foods, like beetroot or certain drugs, can also make your urine change colour. A heavy workout can cause the urine to look red. It's not actually blood, but if it happens while you're exercising or keeps happening you should see your doctor.

If it is blood and it keeps appearing in your urine, it could be caused by an infection of the urinary tract or it could be the sign of something more serious such as a prostate problem. See your GP and try to take a urine sample.

I know condoms are best but it just doesn't feel so good

Not all men are boasting when they say condoms are too tight. Sheaths do vary considerably in size and shape (as well as thickness). Widely available condoms vary by over 20 mm in length and by over 10 mm in circumference. They also come in different shapes, thicknesses and even flavours. If you find one type of condom to be uncomfortable, then shop around until you find another that suits you better.

I've got enough kids – should I have a vasectomy?

A vasectomy operation is performed about 90,000 times every year in the UK (40,000 on the NHS or National Health Service). The official line is that it is a routine procedure that is 99.8 per cent effective for preventing pregnancy and after which the vast majority of men enjoy the same sex life as before.

I'm not sure whether that's true. As editor of <malehealth .co.uk>, I've had more e-mails about vasectomy than about anything else other than penis problems. Most of them complain of post-vasectomy pain (PVP) and poor or no erections.

In the operation, the vas deferens (the two tubes that carry sperm from the testicles) are cut and sealed. It could be that the sperm, which has nowhere to go after this, builds up and causes swelling and pain. It's not quite clear what's going on, but there are signs that the official line is changing. When I wrote an article about this in 2006 I checked the advice on the NHS Direct website. It said that, 'There are no known long-term risks from a vasectomy.' It doesn't say that now.

If you're considering a vasectomy, I'd check out what other men say about it on <malehealth.co.uk>.

3

Beyond the basics: the lazy man's troubleshooting guide

This section of the book deals in more detail with the areas of health that affect us, particularly work, food, drink and exercise. I've called them the 'lazy man's guide' because, frankly, there's very little in here that actually requires you to make major changes. It's about the approach.

How do you spend your day? Roughly like this I should imagine:

- sleeping: 7–8 hours
- working: 7–10 hours
- eating/drinking: 2 hours
- travel: 1–3 hours
- cooking/housework: 1 hour (although your partner probably does much more than this and you probably do less!)
- leisure (exercise, going out, watching TV or reading): 3–5 hours
- sex: five minutes to half an hour.

So what are the health conclusions we can draw from this? Well, it suggests to me that if we can sleep healthily and work healthily, we'll be well on the way to a healthy lifestyle.

Take sleeping healthily. It is not, on the face of it, very difficult. Most of us know what it involves. It's about getting the amount of quality sleep that you need regularly, but the devil is in the detail. What's the right amount for you? How do you make sure it's good quality and regular when life is so busy and stressful?

Of course, there are several practical things you can do to improve your chances of getting a good night's sleep and we'll talk about them on p. 112, but the biggest factor by far is your state of mind. If you're relaxed, happy and pleasantly tired you'll sleep. We all know that. The key is how do you make sure you're relaxed, happy and pleasantly tired at bedtime?

I can't pretend I have a precise answer to that for you (and neither can anyone else except you), but I can tell you what the answer is about. It's about what's between your ears. It's about how you feel about things. Of course, there's an important physical dimension, but basically it's a mental thing. It's in your head.

To a large extent the same is true of work. Most of the things that happen to us at work are not in our control. They're down to colleagues or customers or clients or even bigger, external factors – social and global forces. I was writing this book against the backdrop of a credit crunch, international tension and speculation, which saw the world's financial system in meltdown and left even the most powerful being buffeted around like houses in a hurricane. This is proof, if anyone still needed it, that the only thing you can really control at work is how you react to what happens around you. In other words, it's in your head.

Health isn't about jogging every day or eating tons of vegetables, or even about giving up smoking – although all of these things will help. It's about feeling comfortable in your own skin. Being content within yourself will considerably reduce your chances of having heart attacks, cancer or other major health problems. If – and when – you are affected by them, this sense of being relaxed within yourself will help you to cope with them a lot better than you would have otherwise. In the meantime, you'll get a lot more out of life.

That is why this is the lazy man's troubleshooting guide. Good health is inside your head. You don't have to go anywhere near a gym unless you want to – promise!

Eating: want weight loss without great loss?

Should I go on a diet?

Want to lose weight or eat more healthily? As most men know, diets with a capital D are not your best bet. Diets involving meal replacements, faddy dishes or eating routines usually start well enough but they don't tend to last and they rarely solve the problem. Indeed, many dieters finish off fatter than they started.

The evidence is clear. In 2007, following a review of 31 different studies on this topic, researchers at the University of California concluded that although weight was usually lost during the first six months of a diet, two-thirds of dieters put it back on again – and more – within five years.

To make matters worse, yo-yo dieting – where body weight repeatedly rises and falls – can be more unhealthy than just being a bit tubby. (If you insist on yo-yo dieting, be sure to remove the string first.)

Most diets appear to help at first simply because they force the dieter to think about what he's eating, but they don't last. To some extent, it's down to simple biology. When you start starving your body of calories, it thinks there's a famine and starts laying down as much fat as possible – exactly the opposite of what you want.

Moreover, diets don't work because they don't deal with the underlying problem: our attitude to food. Men who try to lose weight tend to do so not because they want to get into a size zero dress (although if you do the advice here still holds) but because they want to feel healthier. Clearly, cutting down on booze and exercising more will help – and there's more on these elsewhere in this book – but if you want to do it *without* actually changing what you eat, it comes down to two things: go slow and get fresh.

The size of the problem

Being too heavy increases your health risk.

- Obese men are 33 per cent more likely to die from cancer than men of healthy weight.
- A man who is two stone (about 13 kg) overweight is twice as likely to have a heart attack as a man of healthy weight.

About one in four men and women are obese. This is double the level in the early 1990s. Some politicians and health campaigners now talk about an obesity 'epidemic', but let's keep it in perspective. Obesity may be up but the number of men who are overweight – two in five – has stayed pretty much the same.

What's your BMI (body mass index)?

Do you know your BMI? A lot of the discussion of weight is based on this so it's worth knowing yours. Here's the maths:

- BMI = your weight (in kilograms) divided by your height (in metres) squared
- BMI = weight (kg) / [height (m) × height (m)].

Example: For a height of five feet and ten inches (1.78 m) and weight of 13 stone (82 kg), BMI = 82 / (1.78 × 1.78) = 26. Compare this figure with the following BMI categories:

- Less than 20 = underweight
- 20–24.9 = healthy weight range
- 25–29.9 = overweight
- 30–39.9 = obese
- 40 or more = very obese (your health is at serious risk – seek medical advice).

Does all this maths seem like too much hassle? Just measure your waist. If it's over 37 inches (94 cm), then you're probably overweight; if it's over 40 inches (102 cm) then you're probably obese.

What do you mean 'go slow' – take a longer lunch?

That would be a good idea. The point is not to rush your food. To start, don't even think about what you eat. Think about *how* you eat it. Lots of us stuff our faces in front of the telly hardly noticing what we're shovelling in. This is no good.

Take it easy. Drink some water. Look at your food. Chew it. Savour the flavour. Drink some more water. You'll enjoy your food more and your body will know that it's actually eating. This is vital because when it comes to food your brain's a bit slow. It takes it a good 20 minutes to wise up that your stomach is full. This means that if you've been stuffing yourself, you'll have eaten tons more than you wanted.

A good rule of thumb? The first belch. It's dear old Mother Nature's way of telling you've had enough. (And, of course, like all mothers, she does it in the most publicly embarrassing way possible.)

And 'get fresh'?

Once you're eating more slowly you'll taste your food better, so the smart next step is to choose the tastiest version of it.

Now, I'm no farmer but it's clear that the carrot that tastes most like a carrot will be the one you've pulled out of the ground yourself, rather than the one that was picked weeks ago and has since been flown round the world, sliced up, salted, sugared and tinned. The good news is that this fresher version is also the most nutritious version with the most vitamins.

So don't change what you eat but choose the least processed version of it. The more factories and other places your food has been through, the more likely it is to have had sugars, salt and fats added. Avoid ready meals and convenience prepacked options.

Don't buy a chicken meal; buy a chicken instead. When it comes to fruit and veg, frozen is better than tinned, fresh is better than frozen, and organic is better than supermarket.

That is not to say that all fresh food is all that fresh. If the item has been flown from the other side of the world then it's likely to be less fresh than something produced down the road. Check out the country of origin of fruit and veg and buy local.

It's not brain surgery. Baked beans are a good example of the problem with processing. The beans themselves are pretty good for you but in the tins we buy they're pumped up with salt and sugar. Nobody's suggesting you bake your own beans – although you could choose a reduced salt and sugar version – but you see the point.

Apart from the reduction in nutrients, processed foods – and fast foods like burgers and fries too – have a high energy density. That means that each mouthful contains a lot of calories – more calories than your body is expecting.

Human beings have evolved over thousands of years to guess how much we need to eat by the size of a portion, but just an ordinary looking portion of a high-density food can contain double the calories your body expects. If you also have the habit of putting it away like a wolf in a meat factory, you can see how the calories can mount very quickly.

Worst of all, you can become dependent on the sweet, salty, fatty tastes because they give you an instant sugar hit. In tests, rats that are used to this sort of food get the shakes when they're deprived of it. Trouble is that the hit soon wears off and you're back starving again. Now, if only you'd eaten more slowly in the first place. Just like mamma used to say.

How much sugar and salt *can* you eat?

You shouldn't eat more than about a teaspoon of salt a day in total. Too much can raise your blood pressure, tripling your risk of heart disease or stroke.

But that doesn't mean you can sprinkle a whole spoonful on your chips. Far from it. In fact, about three-quarters of the salt we eat every day is *already* in the food, so try to avoid adding any salt at all if you can.

On food labels, check out the amount of sodium per 100 g. (You'll remember from your science lessons that the chemical name of salt is sodium chloride.) Over 0.5 g of sodium per 100 g is high and best avoided. Aim for 0.1 g or 'no added salt'.

The advice is similar with sugar. Don't add it if you can help it, and check the labels. Look for the 'Carbohydrates (of which sugars)' figure on the packet. Choose low sugar (5 g sugars or less per 100 g) or 'no added sugar'.

However, you can deftly sidestep all this hassle if you follow the advice above and avoid processed food as much as possible, especially ready meals (high in salt) and fizzy drinks (high in sugar).

Are you saying the way we eat is not natural?

In a way, yes. Take the idea of evolution a little further and think about the foods we have evolved to eat rather than what we actually eat. Humans like us have been on Earth for at least 200,000 years and 'homo' (human) species very similar to us for at least two million years. In terms of our evolution, the cultivation of crops only began yesterday and the processing of food even more recently.

That's why you hear people going on about the raw food diet or the caveman diet. Sure, they're trying to sell diet books, but the basic theory is sound. For most of our time on this planet, we have been eating what we could hunt and what we could gather from the landscape around us. That means a diet of mainly fruit, nuts, vegetables and meat.

This is not to say that the meat would be much like today's meat. The meat on a hunted animal is different from the flab on a factory-farmed one that has never seen daylight and never walked more than a yard or two. Lean meat, free range, organic or game is closer to what you're after.

So, it's OK to eat meat?

Yes. Meat has been demonized over the years by vegetarians on one side and the cholesterol-lowering industry on the other, but this sort of meat – good quality meat – is good for you, in moderation (twice a week). The real bad boys are not saturated fats – the sort of fat you get in meat – but trans fats.

Indeed, too little saturated fat is linked with depression, tiredness and poor concentration. Lack of vitamin B_{12} causes much the same thing. Because B_{12} is found only in meat, eggs, milk and shellfish, many vegans take a supplement.

What are trans fats?

They're an industrial product created when vegetable oils are converted into something solid and 'spreadable'. They give products a realistic feel when you put them in your mouth as well as a longer shelf-life.

The UK food industry is trying to wean itself off trans fats but you still need to look out for them in margarines, baked products, cereals, fried foods, sweets, chocolate products, spreads, soups, salad dressings, snacks, ice cream and frozen breaded products. (Look for words like 'hydrogenated', 'shortening' and, of course, 'trans' on the food labels.)

What about fish? I've heard that fatty fish is good for you but I thought fat was bad

There are several types of fat, including trans fats (which are best avoided), saturated fats (which we need a little of) and unsaturated fats. The latter are the most healthy and can reduce cholesterol. As well as oily (or fatty) fish, sources include (unsalted) nuts, seeds, oils such as sunflower, rapeseed and olive, and avocados.

The fats in oily fish such as omega-3 are called essential fatty acids. They're essential because the body can't make them itself so we need to get them from our diet. Omega-3s are found in salmon, trout, mackerel, herring, sardines, pilchards, whitebait, tuna (fresh not tinned) and anchovies.

White fish like cod, haddock, plaice and sea bass, while good for you because they're low in unhealthy fats, don't contain as many omega-3s. If you fancy some fish, poach, bake or grill it rather than deep fry it. However, the Food Standards Agency recommends no more than four portions of oily fish a week because these fish can contain pollutants like mercury, especially those near the top of the food chain like swordfish or shark.

As far as omega-3s in meat are concerned, grass-fed meat and dairy products are better choices than grain-fed ones.

What are anti-oxidants?

Anti-oxidants cancel out the cell-damaging effects of so-called free radicals by binding with them.

Free radicals are atoms, molecules or ions that have a spare electron and so are looking around desperately for other free electrons to get together with. It is better that they do this with an anti-oxidant than with your DNA, because the latter could cause cancer. That's the theory anyway. See Table 1 overleaf for a summary of foods rich in anti-oxidants and their benefits; the table also includes other foods that provide important nutrients that are beneficial to your health.

If cereal is so new in our diet, does that mean it's bad for you?

Not at all, but you should try to get the version of the cereal or crop that's closest to nature. That means whole grain or wild rice, and fresh brown bread rather than factory white.

If you're having trouble eating the Government's recommended five portions of fruit and veg a day, you'll find it a lot easier if you replace one serving of cereals, bread, pasta or rice with one of vegetables.

Table 1 Top ten healthy foods (and their benefits)

Food	Rich in	Benefits	Calories/ 100 g	Additional information
Broccoli	Anti-oxidants (betacarotene, vitamins C and E), B vitamins, calcium, iron and zinc	Protects against cancer, heart disease, stroke and cataracts. Has antibiotic properties	33	The Freddie Flintoff of vegetables – a great all rounder
Carrots	The richest source of betacarotene	As above, but also good for liver and kidneys	30	Try sweet potato too
Pineapple	Vitamin C you know about, but pineapple is also a major source of bromlein enzymes	Bromlein enzymes may ease inflammation, aid digestion and reduce blood clotting	41	Pineapple juice is not dissimilar to stomach acid so it's not great for your teeth
Garlic	A natural antibiotic – the king of healing foods	Reduces raised blood cholesterol and lowers blood pressure	100 (one clove equals about 4 g, so unless you're hanging out with a lot of vampires you won't be eating 100 g)	For best results, scoff fresh garlic as soon as possible after chopping. (Pickled garlic is a less smelly alternative)
Ginger	Natural prevention for travel sickness and other nausea	Prevents flatulence, reduces blood clotting, fights colds and may ease inflammation	40	Both garlic and ginger are said to be good for your sex drive

Food	Rich in	Benefits	Calories/ 100 g	Additional information
Oats	Oats are always unrefined, so that they retain their natural nutritional properties. Good sources of B vitamins and fibre	Good for body tissue and can lower raised blood cholesterol, relax the nerves and aid digestion	380	Get your oats but not too often – more than a bowl a day may limit absorption of essential minerals like calcium, iron and zinc
Walnuts	Top non-animal source of omega-3 fatty acids	Good for the heart and with anti-inflammatory properties	720	Provide a good morning boost to the metabolism
Sunflower seeds	These are the top source of the anti-oxidizing vitamin E	Vitamin E tackles free radicals, which are implicated in heart disease, cancer and sports injuries. Pectin removes toxins	600	Two tablespoons (28 g) daily will double most people's vitamin E intake. Another good seed for men is pumpkin
Chilli	Vitamin C and betacarotene	Boosts calorie burning and aids digestion, stimulates body's airways and reduces blood clotting	30 (one chilli equals about 10 g)	Capsain makes chillis hot – most of it's in the seeds. Don't touch your eyes after chopping!
Tea	Anti-oxidants called flavonoids plus fluoride, which protects the teeth. Choose lighter tea (oolong, green, jasmine) for maximum benefits	Lowers cholesterol and blood pressure, protecting against cancer and heart disease	Close to zero (although milk adds a few calories *and* reduces the benefits)	Tea with a meal reduces iron absorption

What, like a large portion of fries?

Potatoes don't really count as a vegetable. Because they're pretty disgusting raw (most of their plant relatives are poisonous), we didn't start eating them in quantities until we learned to cook food. Again this happened relatively recently. In other words, they're not really part of your natural diet any more than the white bread the burger comes in. There's that and the 50 g of fat in a portion of fries.

I've tried all this slow, fresh stuff but I'm still piling on the pounds

I have something for you to try for a while. It is the easiest dietary change that I've come across and one of the few that works.

Prepare and cook your food in the same way and in the same quantity as usual, exactly as described above, but only serve half. Put the rest in the freezer compartment for another time. You'll get all your usual nutrients, just fewer calories. Halving your evening meal will see you losing about two pounds a week. Drink a glass of water ten minutes before you eat to take the edge off your appetite.

That's it. Doddle, isn't it? Eat in halves. If you can drink in them too, so much the better.

Alcohol: when does serious drinking become dangerous drinking?

People drink alcohol in nearly every country on our planet and have been doing so for a long time. Most people do it. Most people enjoy it. Even the Greek philosopher Plato said it was 'a wise man who invented beer'. This makes alcohol probably the most popular drug in the world. Like any other drug, if you're going to take it you need to know how it works.

At its best, alcohol can be part of the fun of being with other people. At its worst it can kill. Worldwide, alcohol kills about nine times as many people as illegal drugs like heroin. Part of knowing how it works is knowing that anyone at any time could develop a problem with alcohol, including you.

The trouble is that we don't quite understand alcohol, especially when we're drinking it. It is true that it helps you to relax. One drink may well help you to relax at a party so that you have more fun, but that doesn't mean that you'll have twice as much fun if you have two drinks. Alcohol encourages you to forget this fact.

Drunk on statistics

More people die from alcohol than heroin. Does that mean that alcohol is more dangerous than heroin?

No. It's an example of how statistics can be misleading. Far fewer people take illegal drugs like heroin than take legal ones like alcohol, but a far greater proportion of the people who take heroin die than those who take alcohol.

When it comes to health, absolute risk is what you should be most interested in, but relative risk – because it's more dramatic – is what is usually reported in the media. For example, say you have a one in ten million chance of catching X. Research shows that drinking tea doubles your chance of catching X. This creates a great headline – 'Tea drinkers at twice the risk of X', but what does it really mean? Doubling the risk means that the chance is two in ten million or one in five million. In other words, although the relative risk has doubled, the absolute risk is still very, very small.

The absolute risk of taking alcohol is far lower than the absolute risk of taking heroin, cocaine or anything else along that line.

What do you mean by one drink? How do you know how much alcohol is in a drink?

Alcohol is measured in units. A unit is eight to ten millilitres of alcohol, which is about two teaspoonfuls. To make life a little easier, the standard drinks sold in bars may all be different sizes but they usually have about one unit of alcohol in them. One unit = one 30 ml glass of spirit (a single measure) = one 100 ml glass of wine = half a pint of ordinary bitter.

Information on units of alcohol is not always user-friendly. Most bottles and tins tell you on the side of them how much alcohol is inside. You can – if you have a degree in advanced mathematics – work out from this how much alcohol you are actually drinking.

For example, say you have a 33 cl (centilitre) can of beer, which contains five per cent alcohol. This 33 cl equals 330 ml (millilitre), so you multiply 330 by 0.05. This equals about 16. This means that there is 16 ml of alcohol in the can, which is about two units.

To add to the confusion, even drinks that are of the same type come in different strengths. A light Australian or American beer may be three per cent alcohol or less. A typical European lager is more like six per cent. Watch out for glass sizes too. These days, large glasses of wine are often close to a third of a bottle, or two to three units.

What does the body do with alcohol?

Like anything you eat or drink, booze goes down your throat and into your stomach. However, while most food stays there to be broken down by the stomach, alcohol doesn't. Alcohol is all over you like a rash.

Thirty seconds after your first sip it reaches the brain. Here it slows down the messages your brain sends to the rest of your body. You feel more relaxed but already it means that there are some things you will find more difficult to do, such as driving, riding a bike, operating machinery or answering questions in the pub quiz.

Full stomach or empty stomach, you'll still be affected. You may notice the alcohol more quickly if you drink on an empty stomach, while a full stomach may mean that the alcohol goes into the blood more slowly, but in the end it's the same story. You get drunk.

So if not in the stomach, where is alcohol broken down?

In the liver. It takes the liver about two hours to break down one unit of alcohol fully. That means that after two hours, the alcohol will no longer affect you, *unless* (and it's a very big unless) you've had another drink.

If you do have another one, your liver then has to start processing this one while it's still working on the other one. Keep drinking and it gets slower and slower, like a computer processor with too many tasks. Meanwhile, your blood alcohol level continues to rise.

The liver doesn't like this much, right?

It's not wild about it, no. Even after just a few drinks, your liver can feel tender and painful the next day.

Here are two facts: liver disease kills ten times as many heavy drinkers as non-drinkers and 80 per cent of liver disease is caused by alcohol. In parts of the UK the number of people getting liver disease has doubled in the past ten years.

Put simply, alcohol kills liver cells making the liver fatty and inflamed. This can cause hepatitis. If you have hepatitis and carry on drinking, the damage becomes irreversible. The disease is then called cirrhosis, and cirrhosis kills.

Liver disease does some other strange things to you too, including disrupting the body's hormones so that you grow breasts and lose hair. If you have liver disease, stop drinking.

OK, since we're into the gory details, how does it affect other parts of the body?

Alcohol slows the brain down sooner and for longer than we think. We often begin to make mistakes that we don't even notice after a unit or less. The brain is still slower the next day. (This is possibly because even if you think you've slept well, alcohol affects your natural sleep patterns.) This is a double problem because when the brain is affected by alcohol it both makes more mistakes and becomes less likely to notice them. We also know that drink can make you depressed.

As for other parts of the body, too much alcohol can cause heart disease and high blood pressure. It can cause stomach problems such as ulcers and cancers of the throat, mouth and tongue. Alcohol is also fattening. (It's made from sugar, remember.) A pint of beer contains about 185 calories – 30 calories more than a 28 g packet of crisps. Alcohol also makes you feel hungry. Put the two together and what have you got? The beer belly or, to put it another way, fat in the most dangerous place for heart disease.

Last but not least, there's sex. Alcohol increases desire but reduces performance. It can make erections poorer. This is both because of the effect of alcohol on the brain – where erections begin – and on blood flow into the penis. In practice, while one drink might help you to get an erection, several won't and with heavy, long-term drinking erectile dysfunction can become regular. Longer term, heavy boozing can shrink your testicles and lower sperm count.

Perhaps this is all just nature's way of preventing us from doing something we might regret in the morning. (A recent study in Bristol showed that 'beer goggles' do exist – even after one unit of alcohol we find people more sexually attractive.)

Tell me about it – alcohol can make you do some pretty stupid things

There's a lot in the book about risk-taking, and alcohol can encourage it in a big way. Most of the time it's nothing serious, but it can be.

In Europe, drunk drivers kill 10,000 people every year. That's more than one death per hour. The British Medical Association has called on the UK to follow the lead of most other European countries and reduce the legal blood alcohol limit for driving from 80 mg per 100 ml to 50 mg. The doctors cite research showing that with 50 mg/100 ml in your blood you're twice as likely to crash as with zero, and ten times as likely to crash with 80.

It's more difficult to get hard and fast crime figures but we know alcohol is a factor in many break-ins, muggings and sex offences. According to the British Crime Survey of 2007–2008, offenders are under the influence of alcohol in the majority of violent crimes, certainly where the victim and offender don't know each other. Alcohol is also behind two out of five incidents of domestic violence.

Heavy drinkers are far more likely to commit suicide than the general population, with alcohol involved in as many as two out of three suicides. If you're drinking because you're unhappy, ask for help. Read the section 'Depression: as dangerous as smoking?', on p. 77.

What are safe levels of alcohol?

The official advice is that men over 21 should drink no more than three to four units a day. Younger men should probably drink less. You should also avoid drinking a couple of days a week and avoid binge drinking (defined as more than six units in six hours). These are the guidelines, but some people may have problems even when they stick to them.

We're all differently affected by alcohol. Your size and metabolism make a difference. So does the time of day and the reason why you're choosing to have a drink in the first place. Don't start drinking if you're already feeling depressed.

The effect of alcohol also depends on age. For people over 45, a couple of glasses of wine a day appears to be good for health. For people under 20 this is not so. What's more, binge drinking is especially dangerous when you're young because your still developing brain is more sensitive.

Moreover, the risk of alcohol is increased if you mix it with other drugs – legal or illegal. If you're on medication, check with your GP how much you can drink.

What causes a hangover?

Alcohol makes you pee, reducing the amount of water in your brain and body, causing headaches. It disrupts your sleep and, of course, your stomach and liver. Add these up and you have that familiar morning-after feeling. Drinking water before going to bed may help make the hangover less unpleasant.

What are the warning signs of a drink problem?

They do vary. Some people with problems with alcohol are very good at hiding it from both other people and themselves. After all, alcoholism is a disease that tells you that you don't have it. If you're worried about yourself, then that alone should be warning enough to cut down and, if you can't cut down, to stop. Check out the section on addiction below, and especially the symptoms of addiction; read Richard's story on p. 74.

There's no shame to having no control over alcohol. Some people have brown eyes. Some people can run fast. Some people have no control over alcohol. It's just the way you are. Throughout this book I've talked about building good health into your everyday life. You can't do that with alcohol problems. If the booze is boss, you need to stop. Because alcohol use is so widespread in our society, admitting that you have no control over it is perhaps the toughest call you'll ever have to make, but if you don't alcohol will kill you.

An early warning sign that you might be at risk is if you get drunk very easily and/or have memory blackouts when you drink and can't remember what happened.

Any tips for cutting down?

- Keep a drink diary – just seeing it in black and white can help.
- Don't get into big rounds or drinking schools.
- Have a soft drink every so often.
- Give up drink for a week, a month, the summer or until Spurs' next win away.
- Say 'no' from time to time.
- Avoid mixing drinks.
- Always know how much you've drunk.
- Limit yourself to spending a certain amount of money.
- Read the sections on depression and addiction in this chapter below.

If you can't do these things, then you don't need to cut down, you need to stop.

Exercise: want to get back in the game?

There comes a time in every man's life when he realizes that if he doesn't start exercising again now he probably never will. One Christmas you'll notice that the weight isn't going away afterwards. Perhaps you'll be breathless after climbing stairs. Whatever the cause, one day it will happen to you.

The vast majority of men do a little or even a lot of sport when they're younger but then let it tail off as careers and families become more important. When this happens, this is the section of the book you need to read.

The good news is that it's not difficult to get back into the exercise game. Indeed, it is easier than you think. It shouldn't even be hard physical work. I told a physiotherapist I know that I was writing this book and he said, 'Men's health is not an intensive sport.' I asked him what he meant and he told me about all the men he'd had in his clinic who'd made the same simple mistake of assuming that they could exercise in the same way at 40 or 50 as they could at 20. He told me the fittest retired guys he knew didn't play sport at all, and some never had – they simply did a gentle 20-minute workout every morning.

Is the physiotherapist right?

Most physical disability in older age is caused not by lack of muscle strength or cardiovascular capacity but by lack of flexibility – not being able to stretch or move freely. A short daily stretching and stamina workout – the sort of thing you do when warming up for a sport – will see you in pretty good stead even if you do nothing else. See the box 'How to warm up' for some tips on stretching and preparing for exercise.

If you're out of condition, stretching is where to start. Don't jump straight back into sport. The old saying 'Don't play sport to get fit, get fit to play sport' is, alas, true. My physiotherapist's litany of busted knees and broken hearts is the proof.

You don't have to make big changes. Just build exercise into what you already do. Walk or cycle instead of taking the car. Get off the bus or train a stop early and walk. Use the stairs instead of the lift. All of these little changes really help. Participants in a study at the University of Geneva saw their chances of premature death reduced by 15 per cent as a result of taking the stairs instead of the lift for just 12 weeks.

How to warm up

Failure to warm up properly is the biggest single cause of sports injury. Most muscles operate in pairs. One muscle contracts as the other stretches. If the stretching muscle isn't warm, it might not respond. The result could be a pulled muscle or ligament.

Warm-up stretches prepare joints and muscles for what is to come. They will enable your body to perform at its best and protect it against injuries, aches and stiffness during the game, the following morning and later in life. Warming up provides muscles with the glucose and oxygen they need for maximum efficiency, and as they get warmer they stretch more easily and you can move your joints more safely.

But won't I be knackered before I start?
If you're a bit unfit or just starting exercise it's tempting to skimp on the warm-up to save yourself for the real thing. Don't. If you find yourself sweating like Tom Jones in a sauna within two minutes of starting exercise, this is because your body is trying to respond to the sudden demands being placed upon it. Warming up will stop this.

On the other hand, don't kid yourself that you needn't warm up because you're fit. Quite the opposite. The difference between the professional and the amateur is not the risk of injury but that the pro knows the importance of warming up.

How long will it take?
The more energetic the exercise and the older you are, the longer and more thoroughly you need to warm up. For vigorous sport, the warm-up itself should leave you a little breathless with a light sweat. Twenty minutes is not an uncommon warm-up time for sports like football.

So what do I do?
Relax. Warm up each muscle group then do some specific stretches appropriate to what you're going to be doing.

Make sure that the quadriceps (muscle at the front of the thigh) and the hamstring at the back are loose and warm. Equally important are the adductors on the inside of the thighs by the groin. This is classic groin strain territory – a difficult muscle injury to treat. For the same reason, do some stretches that loosen your neck. Finish off with activity related to the upcoming exercise. A bit of ball juggling before football, say – it might be the only touch you get. Or if you're swimming, stretch your shoulder, back and neck muscles.

Some stretches are best avoided. Letting your head drop back as far it will go or lying on your back and lifting legs back over your head can both damage the neck. Deep knee bends where you squat right down, sit-ups with straight legs and the windmill (touching toes of one foot with the opposite arm while keeping legs straight) are also dangerous.

Can you be more precise?
If you don't know how to warm up for your sport or type of exercise, ask someone who knows, copy them or check it out on a website. Try the six shown in Figure 4 to start. They should be useful for most activities.

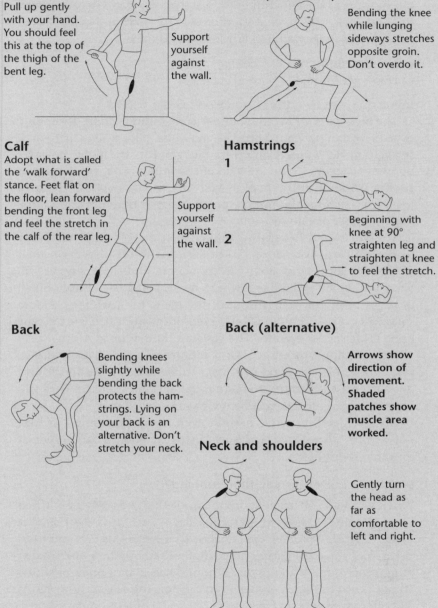

Quads

Pull up gently with your hand. You should feel this at the top of the thigh of the bent leg.

Support yourself against the wall.

Groin (adductors)

Bending the knee while lunging sideways stretches opposite groin. Don't overdo it.

Calf

Adopt what is called the 'walk forward' stance. Feet flat on the floor, lean forward bending the front leg and feel the stretch in the calf of the rear leg.

Support yourself against the wall.

Hamstrings

1

2

Beginning with knee at 90° straighten leg and straighten at knee to feel the stretch.

Back

Bending knees slightly while bending the back protects the hamstrings. Lying on your back is an alternative. Don't stretch your neck.

Back (alternative)

Arrows show direction of movement. Shaded patches show muscle area worked.

Neck and shoulders

Gently turn the head as far as comfortable to left and right.

Figure 4 Some warm-up exercises

What if I want to do something more exciting?

If you want to do something more active, you can find all sorts of tips and advice about what sport or exercise to do and when, but in my experience they all boil down to two things.

• Do something you like doing.
• Don't get injured.

If you do these two things, you won't go far wrong.

The best sport for avoiding injury is swimming. Short of slipping over or picking a fight with the muscular pool attendant, you'll struggle to do yourself anything but good in the pool, however poorly you swim. If you are a decent swimmer, you can get just as good a workout in the pool as you can on the track. An hour of jogging at 5 mph or an hour of gentle freestyle both burn about the same number of calories: 700.

The worst sports for getting injured are contact sports. According to the Football Association, 50 professional footballers have their careers cut short by disability every season, and these guys are fit. Sorry but, much as I'd like it not to be so, going back into football or rugby after you've been out of the game for a while is seldom smart. As every sports fan knows, even the greatest struggle to come back. (This was so even for The Greatest, Muhammad Ali.)

Try standing on one leg for a minute or more. This will give you an idea of how good your core strength is. If you find it very difficult, then do some stretching and specific exercises that will improve your core strength before trying any sports.

However, getting active needn't even involve running – at least not at first. In its way, walking can be as good a fat burner as running, if not better.

Walking is better for you than running?

When you walk, 60 per cent of the calories burned are fat, but when you jog only 40 per cent are. Anita Bean, author of the *Complete Guide To Sports Nutrition*, explained it to me like this: 'As you exercise harder you use a greater proportion of carbohydrate and smaller proportion of fat. Walking for an hour burns 270 calories, of which 60 per cent (160 kcal) comes from fat. Jogging for an hour burns 680 calories, of which 40 per cent (270 kcal) comes from fat. Shorter periods of high intensity exercise will give you the same results in terms of fat loss as longer periods of low intensity exercise.' In other words, walking will get you there in the end.

Walking also means you're highly unlikely to wind up as one of the 25 per cent of people who are forced to give up exercise as a result of their sports injury. These are odds of 4–1, which is a very high risk and one that gets higher the older your body is when you start putting it through its paces.

Point taken: so how do I avoid getting injured?

For those easing back into running or sport, a very useful maxim for ensuring that you remain uninjured is: don't do more today than you will be able to do tomorrow.

It's very easy in a burst of enthusiasm to run too far too quickly, with the result that your legs are battered and aching for days afterwards and you don't go out again. It happens all the time to joggers starting over again.

The typical pattern is this. You take it very easy at first, gradually go a little faster and for a little longer each time, and then on the sixth or seventh run you get injured. The reason is that your cardiovascular performance (your heart and lungs, essentially) rises to the task you're setting for it quicker than your muscles and skeleton.

You notice by the third or fourth run that you're already not so breathless as you were the first time. You're really pleased and rightly so. It's a good sign for your lungs, but it doesn't mean that the rest of your body has improved at the same pace – building up effective muscles takes longer. Pushing them to the new limit that you believe your heart and lungs will allow you to will result in injury.

Why? Because the heart and lungs are brilliantly designed organs. They'll get back to something like their best if you work them properly, but your skeleton won't get stronger anything like as quickly. It will always carry the weight of the past 30, 40, 50 odd years and – if you've a bit of a gut – the weight of the present too.

Your body weight can make a big difference. Depending on how you run and on what surface, you're putting three, four, perhaps six times your body weight through your knee with every step. Over a mile that's 600–800 steps and a lot of weight. So, if you're a big guy to start with you don't even have to be carrying a spare tyre for your body to start to notice.

That needn't be a problem. Your body will tell you all you need to know, but you need to learn how to listen to it. It's very easy – especially for we men who aren't great at listening at the best of times and believe in your that 'no pain, no gain' rubbish – to run through a little aching in legs, especially when your heart appears to be telling you that it's OK. But that pain is there for a reason, and if you ignore it the muscle will give out on you and you won't be running again for a while. At best, it'll be back to square one; at worst you'll join the hordes who drop out of exercise through injury.

To reduce these risks, don't run or do sport every day and especially not at first. Often the after-effects are more noticeable two days after running than the following morning. Taking your time helps you better to get to know your body and how it reacts to what you're putting it through.

Warming up will help, won't it?

Yes. Whatever your chosen exercise, learn how to warm up for it. The normal body temperature is around 37 degrees centigrade, but muscles work best at a temperature of nearer 38.5 degrees centigrade.

Here are some tips and pointers for warming up before exercise.

- Make sure that you're warming up and warming down the right muscles. This is relatively easy with jogging because walking will do it, but for other sports, find out if you're not sure. Any decent website devoted to your chosen activity will tell you – it could make all the difference.
- The older you are the longer you should warm up, and the longer you will be exercising for. This is also true for warming down.
- Warming up and warming down is not just something you have to do so that you can exercise; it is exercise in its own right, because it develops flexibility. Just warming up every day, even if you don't then go on to do anything else, will do you a lot of good.
- If you exercise in the morning, warm up for longer. The muscles are far tighter after a night in bed than after a day in action. In

addition, morning – 10 a.m. to be precise – is the peak time for heart attacks, so take it easy.

Get the right kit (see the box 'How to choose sports shoes'). For most sports this really boils down to decent shoes and – less obviously – the right socks. Most of the rest is just fashion.

Drink a litre of water for each hour of exercise (including swimming), but don't wait until you're sweating to start. Orange squash is a cheap and simple hypotonic drink for before, during and after exercise. (By the way, don't worry about sweating – it's a sign that the body is doing its job.)

How to choose sports shoes

Two out of every three of the UK's recreational sportsmen wear the wrong shoes for their chosen sport, according to Mike O'Neill of the Society of Chiropodists and Podiatrists.

Where should you buy running shoes?
In a specialist shop. A decent shop assistant will be interested in your gait. No, not the thing at the end of your garden but the way you run. They'll help you to answer questions like:

- What's your foot type? You can get an idea by dampening your feet and standing on a sheet of paper. If you can see a full footprint, you have flat feet. If your footprint disappears in the middle to a narrow strip you have high arches. Somewhere in between is normal. A decent assistant will ask about this or even check it out for you.
- Do you over-pronate? You probably don't know but you can tell from looking at your old running shoes, so take them into the shop with you. If the upper leans inwards and the inner sole is well worn on the in-step, then you are probably, er, over prone to over-pronation.

Over-pronation can lead to painful injuries. Flat-footed people are particularly affected. Reducing stride length can help.

Over-pronators need so-called 'motion control' shoes, which have a sturdier, straighter shape (or last) than regular shoes. If you're flat-footed look for multidensity or dual-density midsoles or similar features which are firm rather than heavily padded under the arch.

People with high arches – the least common type of foot – tend to 'supinate' or 'under-pronate'. They generally put a lot of weight on the forefoot, so choose a shoe that is padded here as well as in the heel. A curved (or 'performance') last is better with a high arch. Normal feet tend to prefer a semicurved last.

What about shoes for other sports?
Running shoes are for running in, not for other sports. Again, buy shoes designed for your sport from a specialist sports shop.

For example, racquet sports shoes are heavier and stiffer because racquet sports involve side to side movements and twisting, for which running shoes aren't stable enough. If you want something for activities with a variety of movements such as circuit training or aerobics, try cross-trainers.

Any other tips?
Other points to bear in mind if you want to beat the blisters include the following.

- Feet swell during the day, so buy running shoes in late afternoon or after a workout.
- When laced up there should be about half an inch between your longest toe and the end of the shoe. If in doubt err on the larger side.
- Heel cups should be firm fitting but the insides need to be soft to prevent blisters.
- Go for shock-absorbent soles, especially if you intend to run on the road.
- If you're running on the grass, choose shoes with studs or grooves.
- For hill or fell running, a firmer sole with good support, especially under the arch, is important.
- Replace shoes every 3–6 months or 300–400 miles.
- Try on and walk around in at least four pairs before making your mind up.
- Make sure the top of the heel doesn't rub against your Achilles tendon.
- You might want to learn double loop lacing, which many runners swear makes shoes fit more snugly and better support the arches.

Finally, don't fork out on shoes and then skimp on socks. Choose good quality ones designed for your sport.

How do I know that I'm not doing my old heart more harm than good?

For your heart and muscles to get the most from exercise, the experts reckon that you need to exercise at between 60 per cent and 85 per cent of your maximum heart rate. Working in the 60–85 safe zone ensures that your heart works hard enough to improve it but not so hard that it damages itself. But how do you know if you're in the zone?

Get a heart rate monitor. A basic one is all you need, and they cost no more than a normal watch. This gadget will take account of some of the factors that you might not. Mine showed me how much higher my heart rate was in the morning, for example.

Your maximum heart rate is 220 minus your age, so if you're 40 your maximum heart rate is 220 – 40 = 180 beats per minute. This makes your safe zone a pulse of 108 (60 per cent of 180) to 153 (85 per cent of 180) beats per minute. A heart rate monitor can help you to stay in this zone.

If you're jogging it's easy to follow your heart rate as you exercise. Run until you get out of the zone and then walk until you're comfortably back in it again. It's less easy – but not impossible – with other activities.

Your effective cardiovascular exercise time is the time you spend in this safe zone, not the time you spend running. Time spent walking in the zone is effective too and puts less strain on your muscles and joints. In other words, joggers starting over can happily spend a lot of the time walking and still get the benefit to the heart. Now, tell me that the body is not beautifully designed.

Time spent below the zone is not doing a great deal for your heart and lungs, although it will still exercise your body. Spend too long above the zone and, unless you are an experienced athlete and genuinely fit, you're not doing yourself any favours at all.

Build up your routine slowly. A little more – just a minute more or 50 yards further – is fine. You don't even need to do more each time as long as you're going in the right general direction. Do this without getting injured and you may even start to enjoy it. You certainly won't if you're a hobbling wreck after a week.

Finally, if despite all this you do get injured, follow the advice of Tim Don, four times British triathlon champion. His advice to would-be triathletes is to start with the swimming. 'It's a great way to get fit and of the three disciplines – running, cycling and swimming – it's the one most people don't do as well,' he says. 'If you do get injured doing one discipline you can keep your fitness doing the others. Swimming is a great way to recover after an injury or illness – for everyone, not just professional athletes.' And he should know.

Can you exercise too much?

Yes. Men who burn 2,000–3,000 calories a week through exercise (equivalent to four to five hours of jogging or cycling) have lower death rates than both couch potatoes *and* heavier exercisers (over 3,000 calories/week). Over-exercise results in the production of too much cortisol and boosts circulation of free radicals, which can cause cancer.

How to choose a gym

You don't need to work out at the gym to keep fit, but if you want to go make sure it's a good one. Visit the gym at peak time (6.00–8.30 p.m.) and check out the following.

- Is it overcrowded?
- Is there enough equipment? Does it look clean and well maintained?
- Are machines and free weights in separate areas? (It's best to begin on machines because dropping a dumbbell can be dangerous – especially if you drop it on the big bloke with the 50-inch chest.)
- Are there enough instructors around? Are they qualified? Do they have NVQs (National Vocational Qualifications) in exercise and fitness, for example? Are instructors registered with any professional body? (Ask them.)
- Is there somewhere to warm up and warm down? What are the changing rooms and showers like?
- Don't be over impressed by fancy video screens. Air conditioning, lighting and drinking water facilities are more important. If you do want to watch telly while exercising, check out what's on.
- Check whether the programme of classes suits you.

- Check the fees – these can be harder to work out than a phone bill. Ask whether there is a joining charge or any additional costs for classes or other facilities, and how you cancel or suspend your membership.
- Try it out – before joining get a daily or weekly pass and see what the place is really like.

Good gyms will give new members a fitness assessment. If you haven't exercised for a while, ask for a fuller one from an instructor. Before letting you on the equipment, a good gym will explain how it all works.

What gear do I need for the gym?

Don't buy anything too expensive: a water bottle, two towels (large for the shower and small for wiping sweat off the equipment), toiletries, something to keep sweat out of your eyes (sweatband, bandana or the like), a healthy post-gym snack to deter you from going to the pub or sweet shop, and your gym kit. You can read or listen to music on some machines, so pack your iPod. Weightlifting gloves are also useful for, er, weightlifting.

Work: the twenty-first century's biggest threat to health?

Work is insidious and evil. It gets up the nose and under the skin. It's a dangerous killer and should probably be illegal.

I'm exaggerating a little perhaps, but that's not surprising. In the summer prior to publication of this book (2008), I came back from my nice little holiday to find more than 500 e-mails awaiting my attention. All of the relaxing benefits of revitalizing sunshine, eating properly, swimming regularly, cycling daily and reading a couple of decent books were gone in two clicks of a mouse. 'Just delete the lot,' said a mate.

I never had the nerve to follow that advice. The result? I was back to square one. Behind square one, in fact – not sleeping properly, deadlines, and to-do lists and other work-related crud filling my head. Why did I need a holiday in the first place?

Work is like the washing up – it never ends. So why do we do it?

The answer is not as obvious as it seems, because even people who have plenty of money work. I once interviewed a guy who won £2.3 million on the lottery on Saturday and went back to his job on the railways on the Tuesday. Many professional footballers earn enough in a year or two to last most of us a lifetime, yet no footballer ever retires because he's got enough in the bank and doesn't need to be kicked up in the air by John Terry any more. (At least, none admit it.) The lottery winner said he realized that he enjoyed his job, and I suppose footballers feel the same.

So is it simply that I don't enjoy my job? Clearly, spending eight to ten hours a day doing something that makes you unhappy is pretty damaging to your mental well-being and probably your physical health too, but I don't think it's as simple as that in my case. You're pretty much your own boss as a freelance writer, and most of what I write about is interesting and feels socially useful.

It's more to do with how I – and a lot of men, I think – feel about work. Men in particular identify with their jobs. We become what we do. I like to think of myself as someone who takes everyone as they come and doesn't care about status, but when I'm introduced to a man or woman it's amazing how quickly I ask what he or she does for a living. We classify people according to their work. Can't help it.

So if work is part of how you identify yourself, you need to feel that you're doing it well, and the truth is that in the modern workplace very few people honestly feel that. Whether you're in an office, factory or on site, whether you use a computer or a crowbar, you're constantly trying to get more done in less time. Things usually get done well enough but rarely as well as they could be done.

If that bothers you, then you're in trouble. I imagine this nagging 'not as good as it could be' is even worse in a job like teaching or caring, but the people who sleep with their smartphone under their pillow know this feeling too. In other words, if you like your job you probably can't do it as well as you'd wish to. That's bad for your health. If you don't like your job, then you spend eight to ten hours each day doing something that makes you unhappy, and that's bad for your health too.

Aren't you exaggerating? A lot of people enjoy their work

Yes, perhaps I am exaggerating, but not by much. In 2007 an incredible 36 million working days were lost in the UK to work-related ill health and injury – that's one and a half days for every single worker. At least 241 workers were killed at work, and well over two million people were suffering from an illness caused or made worse by work. The Japanese even have a word for 'death from over-work' – *karoshi*. In 2007, the Japanese Government published its highest karoshi figures ever.

The workplace is not likely to get any healthier in the near future. We're working longer hours. In 2008, some 3.3 million people in the UK were working more than 48 hours a week. (Between 1998 and 2006, the number of people working more than 48 hours actually went down from 3.8 million to 3.1 million.)

Cary Cooper, Professor of Organizational Psychology and Health at UMIST (University of Manchester Institute of Science and Technology), says that research internationally shows time and again that there is a relationship between long hours and ill health, even if you choose to work long hours. 'Work 35–40 hours a week for 50 years and you're probably going to be all right. Go consistently over 41 hours a week and you will damage your health and reduce your working life.'

Long hours are the only way to make enough money

If all of these extra hours are mostly for money, then most of us are getting less than our fair share. According to the Joseph Rowntree Foundation, the gap between rich and poor in Britain is wider than it has been for more than 40 years. Social mobility, as the sociologists call it, is down. Children born poor in the 1950s had more chance of becoming rich than those born poor in the 1970s.

It used to be that there were compensations for relatively low pay – job security (you might not earn much but at least you knew it would continue), good pensions and other perks. But all this has gone too. Outsourcing, freelancing and contracting – coupled with the reduced influence of the trade unions – has put an end to job security.

Even if you still have a pension, it could well be next to useless. Pension apartheid is the way ahead, with a dwindling number of older hands on decent defined benefit schemes and newer recruits stuck with defined contributions but no idea what the benefits will be.

All this adds to work stress. (Even more so, following the economic crisis of late 2008 that was exploding as I was writing this chapter.)

Finally, if low pay, long hours and reduced job security at a time of falling house prices and spiralling food and energy costs isn't enough to keep you awake all night with the screaming ab-dabs, the job – for all but a handful – is as dull as dishwater.

Modern management is about numbers and targets. 'If you can't measure it, you can't manage it' is the modern management maxim. Twaddle. If your boss can truly only manage numbers, it's his or her management technique that needs restructuring and not the business.

Few of the things that really matter – imagination, innovation, fun, wit, love and laughter – can be measured. Neither, to come back to how much men identify with their work, can self-respect. If none of these things matter in today's workplaces, no wonder so many of them are such unhealthy places to be.

You've obviously had some pretty bad bosses

It is not just me that thinks this – Businesslink, the Government-backed business support service, agrees. They advise on the most common causes of stress at work. All but one of them are related to bad management:

- high workloads
- lack of control
- lack of support
- inadequate training
- a blame culture
- weak management
- multiple reporting lines
- poor communication.

The other main contributor to work-related stress is an unhealthy working environment.

If work is so dangerous then what can I do about it?

Know the law. Under health and safety law, although your boss is responsible for making sure you are safe at work, so are you. If you don't follow safety regulations and have an accident, it may be your fault. Ask about safety if you're not told, and remember – you can refuse to do something that you think is dangerous. Look out for the health and safety poster in your office. Under the law, your boss must have one on display. There should also be information on fire, accident, first aid, and any other health and safety arrangements. Make sure you know who in your office is trained in first aid.

The two organizations in charge of making sure your boss is following the rules are the HSE (Health and Safety Executive), which looks after factories, farms and building sites, and your local council, which looks after offices, shops, hotels and catering and leisure activities.

If you have any health problem, illness or disability that affects the way you do your job, then your employer may well be obliged by the Disability Discrimination Act to help you with it. Remember, you don't have to consider yourself disabled or have any special pass or claim any particular benefit to be covered. Under the law, your employer must make any 'reasonable adjustment' that will enable you to do the job despite your health problem. What was once high-tech is now mainstream, and you'll be amazed by how many adjustments are possible.

Your employer is obliged to carry out a risk assessment on any equipment you use, including a computer. You don't need to be old or doing the job for a long time to get RSI (repetitive strain injury). In fact, young people are more likely to be working in environments and jobs that put them at risk of RSI, so watch out. As well as a safe work station, you also have the right to eye tests and breaks.

Who can help me with this?

The best source for all information on your rights at work is a trade union. It's your legal right to join one.

What can I do myself to make my own working environment healthier?

Health hazards lurk around every corner in most offices, and I don't just mean the boss. Don't underestimate the damage a badly designed workplace can do. About half a million UK workers have RSI in their arms and wrists. I have an RSI that still comes back from time to time. At its worst it was so bad that I couldn't work. At one point I wondered whether I'd ever work normally again and had to negotiate my own redundancy. This was very stressful. It happened just a year or so before I got cancer, and I've always thought that it was part of the cause.

Most RSI cases are among computer users, and a major cause is a poorly designed keyboard and mouse. You can avoid RSI by:

- keeping your hands warm
- taking frequent breaks (at least once every 15 minutes)
- doing lots of gentle neck rolls and hand and arm stretches
- setting your work (or play) station up so your elbows are at right angles and the screen is at eye level
- learning keyboard shortcuts so you aren't over-dependent on the mouse
- knowing the law – employers have a legal obligation to provide safe computer work stations.

Today there are many keyboards and mouse designs that are more user-friendly. Check them out.

Diabolical desks are the other major contributor to RSI. Desks should be at a height that allows you to sit with your feet flat and your elbows to bend at 90 degrees. Chairs should support your back while you work. Get up from the desk regularly.

By the way, frequent driving can cause RSI too. Set up your car seat properly. There should be just a foot between you and the steering wheel. (Most people sit too far back and strain their back.) Use a small cushion to support your lower back and adjust your rear view mirror to keep you sitting upright.

The average office is drowning in electromagnetism from electrical items and radio waves, including TVs, phones and wi-fi. Although we don't know the exact risks these pose, what we do know is that the levels, even from simple electrical cables, are far,

far higher than anything we've evolved to deal with in the natural environment. Some people are sensitive to this and it's probably a big factor in so-called sick building syndrome – offices where people seem always to be coming down with headaches, tiredness, itchy and sore eyes, colds and coughs.

But what can I do about sick building syndrome? I can't knock the office down

The idea is to get your surroundings in the place you work as close to that of the outside environment as you can. Why? Because outdoors is the environment more than 200,000 years of evolution has prepared us for – not the office.

Get some plants. They look nice and help normalize temperature, carbon dioxide and humidity levels. Some absorb the volatile organic compounds produced by photocopiers and printers. Try peace lilies, bamboo palms, Boston ferns, rubber plants, azaleas and tulips.

Lighting can make a big difference to your mood, alertness and sleep. Put a natural lightbulb in your desk lamp and ask the boss to fit full spectrum lighting. Sit by the window. If you sometimes crave to open the window you're possibly ion sensitive (about a third of us are). Ions are electrically charged molecules, and too many positive ones can have negative effects. Because of all of the electrical equipment, the ions in the air of the average office are more positively charged than ladies' nights in Benidorm. Fresh air is a natural source of negative ions. Windows also provide natural light and, if you're lucky, a stimulating view of the gas works.

Offices are often too hot (room temperature should be 16 degrees C according to the HSE) and the air too dry. Workers in air-conditioned offices are far more likely to have breathing problems than those in naturally ventilated environments. If your office temperature is uncontrollable, then wear layers of clothing so that you can control your temperature yourself.

Take real breaks. The brain works in one and a half to two hour concentration cycles throughout the day, so build your breaks around this. When you do stop, do something completely different if you can – go for a walk, listen to music or do some stretches.

Keep a bottle of mineral water on your desk and sip regularly –

it'll keep your intake of the body's natural lubricant up and your consumption of coffee and other stuff down.

Finally, if you can work outside from time to time, do it.

Working in the park is a nice idea but I'm just too busy. How do I avoid stress at work?

You can't. It's how you deal with it that matters. Rather than trying to avoid it or, even worse, denying that it affects you, it's best to learn to let it out. First, learn to recognize your symptoms of stress. Typical warning signs include:

- feeling you're losing control
- thinking about work even when you're not doing it
- problems sleeping or eating
- feeling the need for drink or drugs
- shorter temper
- reduced attention
- inability to focus
- loss of interest in sex, appearance and life in general.

Stress is inevitable in the twenty-first century. There is more information in a single edition of today's newspaper than the average person would come across in a whole lifetime 300 years ago. No wonder we sometimes feel swamped. Don't take things – or yourself – too seriously. Take pride in what you do but don't try to control everything. Change is inevitable and also unpredictable. Don't fight it, enjoy it.

You could prioritize your work by making a daily 'to do' list. Writing things down frees the mind for what it's best at. If you really have too much to do, tell your boss. If you don't feel you can do this, talk to a work mate or your trade union. If there's no union where you work, talk to the TUC (Trades Union Congress) – they have a 'Know your rights' line (0870 600 4882) – and check out their website (<worksmart.org.uk>).

Here are six dead easy stress control techniques.

- Sing. The breath and lung control needed for singing will get you breathing normally and thinking clearly again.
- Swim. Actually, any physical exercise will help but, when you

add the relaxing effect that just looking at water can have, swimming is probably the best bet for stress.

- Have sex. Making love gets the heart and the hormones going, helps you to sleep and reduces irritability. (It's ideal if your stress is caused by time pressure because, according to the famous Kinsey report, 75 per cent of men finish within two minutes.)
- Read. Dive into a book. Whether it's Harry Potter, Wayne Rooney's autobiography or the wisdom of Jeremy Clarkson (quite a short one that), reading in the evening helps relaxation and sleep, and can even ease depression.
- Do nothing. For five minutes a day, sit or lie down, put some music on if you like, but don't actually *do* anything. Relax. (This is not as easy as it sounds but worth it.)
- Think of nothing. Once you've mastered doing nothing you can take it a stage further: lie flat on your back and, working up from your feet, tense each muscle group in turn for about five seconds and then relax them for ten. Move slowly up your body finishing with your face, mouth and eyes. Now relax, concentrating on breathing deeply and enjoying the quietness.

Think you can't do any of these at work? You'd be surprised. The boss has been doing the last one for years.

You say you're busy but are you addicted? Work is one of the many things it's possible to become addicted to. More on this in the following section.

Addiction: how can something that felt so good feel so bad?

We live in a world of plenty. You can get pretty much anything you want whenever you want, one way or another. This means that the problem of too much – even of a good thing – is a problem like never before.

The principle behind addiction is simple. A therapist at one of the famous Priory clinics once explained it to me like this: 'Everyone likes to change the way they feel and when we find something that works for us we obviously go back to it. For some, it gets out of control but the point is that initially an addiction works.'

Drinking, illegal drugs, prescription drugs, gambling, slot machines, sex, porn, masturbation, having affairs, work, the internet, computer games, sport, exercise, smoking, dieting, binging, sugar, shopping, shoplifting – the list of possible addictions goes on. Clearly, some addictions are more serious than others, and some are more likely to kill you than others. However, even seemingly quite harmless addictions – the sort of thing we joke about – can be damaging.

In 2005, the UK had its first case of texting addiction. 'It's kind of comforting when you get a message. It's like a game of ping-pong, as you send one and get one back,' said the teenager who lost his girlfriend, thousands of pounds and his job after sending up to 500 e-mails and texts each day from work.

Yes, there are many activities that some people do quite happily on and off for their whole lives that others, sooner or later, become addicted to. How do you tell the difference?

- Preoccupation – you're thinking about the activity even when you're not doing it. You begin to see people in terms of how they relate to your habit – drug buddies.
- Escalation – you need more to get the same buzz, or you need to do it for longer and longer.
- Cost – your habit is beginning to cost you more than just the cost of the drink, drugs or whatever it is, and is affecting your relationships and family life.
- You've tried to stop or cut down and you can't. You're impatient and easily angered when you can't do it for a while.
- You're lying to others about what exactly it is that you're doing – playing down your drinking or your gambling losses, for example.
- Escape – you're aware that you're doing what you're doing to change the way you feel or avoid something. You're doing it to forget.
- Absorption – you lose track of time when you're doing it.

People often try to draw their own lines in the sand to kid themselves that they don't have a problem – 'I'm OK because I don't drink in the mornings.' 'I'm OK because I don't do drugs at work.' 'I'm OK because I only have a bet at the weekends.'

Then the lines start to move. One day it's, 'I'm OK because I don't do it on a Sunday in a leap year when the moon's in Uranus and West Ham are at home,' but deep inside you know you have a problem (and I don't mean with your football team). Knowing it is easy – the tough bit is admitting it to yourself.

If you can, talking to family and friends might help. It helped Jason (see below), but this is not always easy. Talking to a doctor might be easier. GPs are used to pointing people in the right direction for help with their addiction.

You can also contact groups of other addicts who are on the road to recovery. Alcoholics Anonymous began in the USA in the 1930s. There are now many groups taking a similar approach with other addictions, including gambling, sex and drugs. There are other groups too that a careful internet search will help you to find. (There's more about using the internet for health information in the section 'So what is the internet good for?' in Chapter 4.)

The favourite gag of the recovering addict is that denial is not just a long river in Africa. Denial is the barrier between you and recovering your freedom. Seek help. There is no shame in being an addict, even to something that might disgust or appal you. It could happen to anyone. Here are five men it happened to. You'll find them most useful if, when you read their stories, you think about the similarities with your life and not the differences.

'I thought if I could work harder it would be OK'

Michael

Both my parents were in business working long hours so I never knew any different. Once I started work myself I gradually let every other interest in life go. I loved having a long list of things to do. For the last seven years of my working life I thought about nothing else. At best I was only getting two hours sleep a night, waking up in cold sweats. I had blackouts. I knew something wasn't right but thought that if I could work harder it would be OK.

The GP put me on anti-depressants but that didn't help. When I eventually saw a psychiatrist he admitted me to hospital immediately. I was on suicide watch, being checked every half hour. When the psychiatrist suggested work addiction I thought it was complete nonsense, but as I was powerless over my addiction I knew I had to make a leap of faith if I was to survive.

I followed the programme. Accepting my problem and that I could get well gave me hope and that built into a recovery. Now I do voluntary work talking to other addicts. I encourage people to recognize their similarities with other addicts. Because the work ethic is seen as a positive thing, the addiction creeps up on you. There are a lot of undiagnosed work addicts out there.

'Internet porn was accessible, distracting and appealing'

Jason

I had no interest really in porn before the internet. I went to a fairly strait-laced boys' school so it was passed round as a bit of a currency there. I guess that gave porn a certain mystique, but I never used it after I left school and I wasn't obsessed with sex.

When I got hooked, I was in a relationship that wasn't going anywhere and I was frustrated with my career in information technology. I was bored and web savvy. Internet porn was accessible, distracting and appealing. It was easy to pass the time looking at it. Two hours could pass in a flash. Although there's no physiological addiction to porn as there is to, say, drugs, the state you get into does release soothing brain chemicals that can become addictive. You're almost in a trance, lost in looking. Sexual stimulation is an element, but there are many addicts for whom it goes beyond this. Some men spend all day looking and don't masturbate at all. In fact, they don't want to come as they don't want to break the spell.

The key thing is motivation to change. You need to understand that you have developed this problem for a reason – you're not inadequate, sad or a pervert. It's important to try to identify what the reason is and address it directly. You need to make practical changes. Smokers avoid situations where they might be tempted to smoke. You can avoid solo surfing. It's about recognizing you have choices and giving yourself options. It's also important to recognize that – like the smoker – you may well relapse, but that doesn't mean you're back to square one. You've got all the learning that you've picked up on the way to help you as you give up again.

'I gave him all the clichés about working hard, playing hard'

Richard

At about 21, the warning signs started. I was in a pub with my dad. He said he'd noticed that I'd always had a drink before we met and was drinking quickly and choosing stronger beers. I gave him all the clichés about working hard, playing hard. I absolutely denied there was a problem. From 21 until I stopped at 27, there was hardly ever a day I didn't have a drink. I began putting on weight and I was stammering more than I had as a child. In other words, the booze was beginning to bring back the problems it had previously covered up.

We had a row and my girlfriend screamed at me, 'Richard, you're 25 and you're an alcoholic.' That was the first time anyone had used the word. I used it as an excuse to leave and go to the pub. I wasn't going to admit I was an alcoholic because of the popular perception of one as an old git in rags.

I didn't admit I had a problem until the day I phoned the AA (Alcoholics Anonymous). When I talked to someone on the phone, I realized I wasn't the only one. The London Regional Telephone Service passed my name on to a member of the AA in my area. I agreed very reluctantly to go to a meeting with him the next day. I was nervous in case I was put on the spot. They gave me a cup of tea and suggested I sit and listen and try to identify with the similarities between my experiences and those of others, not the differences. The room was full of people – young, old, both sexes. A cross-section of society. That weekend I went to a meeting every evening and I haven't had a drink since.

'It's like having cancer and treating the hair loss'

Phil

I was a chubby kid and got teased about my weight, which I didn't like. The first time I vomited I must have been about 12. I didn't do it on purpose, I was ill, but I noticed that I lost weight. I started weighing myself twice a day and realized that vomiting could make a difference. I started making myself sick more often.

When I was older I got into drinking and drugs like heroin and cocaine. As the years went by I found that even when I could give these up I could never stop being bulimic. At first I really thought it was the solution. It brought me a peace within myself that I'd never had. But by 27 I was following the same behaviours with regard to food that I had followed with drugs – lying to people, manipulating them, eating to make myself numb. I was back in drugs rehab. I was sick of being sick but I still didn't tell them about the bulimia.

I knew the food didn't do it any more for me but I couldn't live without it. Anything sweet I'd eat. I'd even eat frozen food while it was still frozen. I'd eat standing on the scale and then vomit to see exactly what difference it made. I could see myself vomiting myself to death. I knew I had to stop.

I already knew about the 12 steps programme and that it could work so I got in touch with Overeaters Anonymous and saw a therapist. I started studying and working in a rehab centre. I'm now an addictions counsellor.

Food is the major mood-altering substance in the world today – it's everywhere, totally legal and relatively cheap. About 90 per cent of my private counselling practice is to do with eating disorders. A lot of men are like me – they present with drugs or alcohol problems but there's an underlying eating disorder. It's easier for men to admit to drink or drugs, I think.

The male body is objectified in today's society just as much as women's are and that increases the stress on people with a poor body image. Stress is a key trigger for eating disorders, but weight is just the tip of the iceberg for many. It's like having cancer and treating the hair loss.

I'm actually bigger now than I was at 27 but I'm much happier with myself these days.

'I don't want to stop trading but I'm a compulsive gambler'

Sam

Gambling really took hold of me when I was about 14. A friend introduced me to how to win the jackpot on fruit machines. I won the first time I tried and walked away, but I was hooked – I began to lose small amounts and then try to win it back. Because I was getting through my pocket money in a couple of days I started stealing. I progressed to more expensive machines, sometimes losing quite a lot each day and being full of shame and swearing not to do it but always, always going back for more.

At university I thought I had it licked, but after my first year I went home for the summer and decided I was free now and could use my credit cards to just try my luck at the casino. I managed to go from being in credit by a few hundred pounds to being down by thousands in six weeks.

I had to stop my career path for various reasons, some of which were caused by my gambling and the position it put me in terms of my health and welfare. But I got married to a wonderful woman and have two children now. I paid off my debt and thought I was safe, at least for the moment. But I lost my career path again. I've had a long period out of work which I could officially put down to health issues, but whenever I've felt a bit better I've tried a flutter and it sends me back to the desperation of the hopeless gambler.

I got into a form of financial markets hedging used by big institutions, banks and hedge funds to protect against bad trades in equities and other instruments. I thought I'd found a real career answer. Many times I've traded my account up as much as 300 per cent in a few months through really great trading skill and discipline. But then I get greedy and go for the ultimate win.

I contacted Gamblers Anonymous because I'm losing hundreds per day, and for my and my family's sakes I'm seeking help because it's not my money any more. I really don't want to stop my trading because it does offer an opportunity and I know I have got what it takes, but without some kind of help I'm helpless to avoid being a compulsive gambler with my life. I need a big change.

Depression: as dangerous as smoking?

There probably shouldn't be a separate section on mental health in this book at all. As mentioned at the start of this chapter, all good health is between your ears. In fact, the relationship between what's going on inside our heads and what's going on in the rest of our bodies is so close it's often difficult to tell them apart. Your state of mind will make a difference both to the sort of health challenges you face and how you deal with them.

Depressed men often have low levels of testosterone and high levels of cortisol, the hormone released in response to stress. This combination increases the risk of erection problems, diabetes, cancer and heart disease. In fact, the risk of heart disease is about three times higher in men with a diagnosis of depression. Some experts will go as far as to say that depression causes heart disease just as surely as smoking does. There is also a clear link between mental health problems and cancer. For example, a study of civil servants published in 2008 found that those who had been off work with depression had double the risk of dying of cancer.

What does this mean? It means that if you're angry or depressed, doing something about it won't just make you happier or more relaxed, but it will also reduce your risk of serious diseases.

Mental illness, particularly depression, is behind 90 per cent of suicides. There is a strong family link here. The statistics show that if someone in your family committed suicide then the chance that you will do the same is higher – six times higher if they were a parent or sibling. So if you do have suicide in your family history, it's even more important for you to seek help if you're depressed.

Depression and mental illness present one of the most serious health issues in the world today, but at least half of all cases are undiagnosed and untreated. Can you imagine the outcry if half of the cases of cancer went untreated? Although doctors are taking the condition far more seriously these days, it is still largely down to you to seek help if you think you're affected.

How common is depression?

It is very common. Around 15 to 25 per cent of the UK population experiences depression or anxiety. That's as many as one in four of us. Worldwide, the World Health Organization estimates that depression will be the second biggest cause of death and disability by 2020. In 2006 the Government's advisor on mental health told the Prime Minister that depression, anxiety and other forms of mental illness had overtaken unemployment as the biggest social problem in the UK. He estimated the economic cost at around £17,000,000,000.

What causes depression?

Depression can be triggered by a particular event or by a build-up of events or problems over time. These might include the death of someone close to you, the loss of your job or house, or being the victim of abuse, injustice or violence. They might have happened very recently or many years ago. They can happen to anyone, which means that depression can happen to anyone. There's no shame in it – in fact it's quite normal to feel depressed after some of these things. But different events affect different people in different ways, and in some people they echo and resound in ways that won't go away, causing pain and unhappiness.

I reckon that my personal problems with depression started when I was about 13. I was a bit of a sensitive kid. Now, in general, I believe that sensitivity is a quality worth having but if it is coupled with a lack of knowledge about yourself and the world – a combination found in many kids – it can be dangerous.

I suffered no abuse, no great loss or bereavement. It was just things that happen to umpteen kids every single day around changing school. I am well aware that in the mind of another child these things would probably have had no impact at all, but I also recognize – and this is the point I'm trying to make here – that in the mind of another child the effects might have been worse. We're all different.

We know that smoking will kill half of the people who do it. What we don't know is who. It could be you or it could be your brother. It could be your friend Eric or the guy who works in the chip shop. Who knows? It's the same with depression. We don't know who it will hit or hit hardest. It has nothing to do with mental strength – in fact, what really takes mental strength is to admit to yourself that you're depressed. It took me about 25 years.

How do you know if you're angry or depressed?

This is a good question. When you're depressed you often don't notice anything much, including changes in yourself, so it is possible to drift into depression and not be aware of it. This can last a long time. Some warning signs of depression include:

- feeling tired all the time but not able to sleep;
- loss of interest in the basics like eating, washing, sex or changing clothes;
- staying needlessly late at work;
- excessively or unusually loud behaviour (difficult to spot in some people, admittedly);
- over-the-top reactions like excessive anger, sadness or competitiveness;
- feeling pressured by ordinary everyday events;
- avoiding people and spending lots of time alone;
- feeling like you want to explode or hit something;
- digestive problems or sickness after eating; and
- lack of concentration.

Anger is often the other side of the same coin. You don't have to blow your top every five minutes to have an anger problem. Passive anger can be just as dangerous. Your anger might be causing you longer term mental health problems if:

- you don't get over anger for a long time and find yourself holding grudges;

- you feel ratty and frustrated or disappointed most of the time, even if you don't actually get obviously angry;
- you feel yourself suddenly becoming out of control when you get angry;
- you deliberately hurt others or break things when angry;
- you're drinking or using other drugs to calm yourself down; or
- you take out your anger on someone other than the person who has actually made you angry.

What can help?

Talking can help. If you can talk to your friends, partner or family, so much the better. Even if you can find just one mate you can really talk to, you won't regret it. Many people think that men have fewer friends that women. I'm not sure whether this is true. Men may have fewer in number, but it's quality not quantity that counts here.

Friends can help you to live longer. Put bluntly, older people with good networks of friends are less likely to die. A recent study in Australia put a number on this; people with friends were about 22 per cent less likely to die over the ten years covered by the study than people without. It also suggested that friends were far more important than family in this respect.

The reason for this is probably that friends can be easier to talk to than family. Family are often too involved in your life, especially the formative childhood years, to be objective. They want you to feel better as soon as possible, so they may suggest that you 'do this' or 'do that', when all you really want is to say how you feel. Your partner too may have much invested in a certain view of you and may be uncomfortable with your feelings. Let's be frank about it, boys don't cry for a good reason. That reason is that the people around us – and that often includes our partners – don't like it.

Old friends – mates who have known you since you were young – are increasingly important as you get older. So even if you haven't much in common right now with people you used to know at school or in a previous job, keep in touch with at least some of them. Things will change and your friendship might do you both a favour in the future. The internet makes keeping in touch pretty easy.

It's OK to talk to your friends about everyday problems that will pass but what about deeper stuff?

I agree. Under these circumstances, friends might be sympathetic at first but most of them – understandably – will tire. (Friendships are supposed to be fun, after all.)

It can be very useful to talk to people who don't know you and won't judge you. This could be a group of people – this is exactly how Alcoholics Anonymous and similar groups work, for example – or it could be one person who is a skilled listener. That is where talking therapies come in. 'Talking therapies' is the general term used for counselling, psychotherapy and the other therapies that are based on the simple idea that talking helps. Although talking with a counsellor or other professional may not be for everyone, there are many men who feel it is not for them but who would benefit greatly – me, for example. I was sure that it was things outside me that were making me unhappy. But I came to realize that it was my reaction to them that was causing the real problem. I won't pretend that talking is easy but I can guarantee that it helps. The key thing is to find the right person – or people – to talk to.

There's more on how to talk about the things you can't bear to talk about in the section 'How do I talk about the thing I can't talk about?' on p. 97.

Talking treatments are particularly important for men when it comes to dealing with issues such as depression and anger, because the drugs are less likely to work for us.

What drugs are available?

The drugs most commonly used to treat depression are SSRIs such as Prozac, but they're really for more severe forms of depression. For mild depression, NICE (the National Institute for Health and Clinical Excellence – the Government body that sets the guidelines for NHS treatments) recommends talking treatments and exercise.

Why are these drugs less effective in men?

Only two-thirds of patients respond to SSRIs, even by the most optimistic estimates. SSRIs stands for 'selective serotonin reuptake inhibitors' and, because of the differences between men and women in the way our brains handle the neurotransmitter serotonin, the patients who benefit are more likely to be women than men. Having said that, these anti-depressants can help if they are used under strict medical supervision for more severe depression. That's supervision with a capital 'S', because there is also an increased risk of suicide on SSRIs.

How could an anti-depressant make you kill yourself?

Nobody really knows, and the drug companies don't really want to talk about it. The best explanation I've heard is from men's health expert Marianne Legato of the Gender Specific Medicine Centre at Columbia University. She quotes her father, also a doctor, who believed that as patients begin to recover their risk of suicide increases, because the slight lifting of depression gives them the energy to plan a suicide and carry it out. The fact that the risk of suicide is higher in younger men on SSRIs lends support to this theory.

What about St John's Wort?

In 2008, an expert review analysed 29 different studies of the herbal treatment St John's Wort and found that it could be effective in easing depression and had fewer side effects than SSRIs. However, there are two factors to bear in mind. The strengths of the numerous preparations vary, so make sure you get the right dosage. (The dosage of St John's Wort used in most studies is a 900 mg/day.) St John's Wort can also interfere with some prescription drugs, so get a health professional's advice before using it. Like SSRIs, St John's Wort might take up to six weeks to start working.

Can't I just read a book?

I hope this book helps. On the malehealth website (<malehealth.co.uk>), there are articles on mental well-being by numerous authors, ranging from a psychiatrist who got depression himself to the spin doctor Alastair Campbell. I hope that these help too, but reading about these things can only take you so far.

Forget the psychological self-help books with whacky titles that promise you the world. The material in them may have worked for the author – or may not – but it won't necessarily work for you. Reading self-help books is really just a delaying tactic.

Writing is far more useful than reading. If talking to someone else seems daunting at first, talk to yourself. Things become clearer when you write them down. Writing for nobody's eyes but your own can soothe away those little irritations that combine to drag down your day.

Keep a diary?

It need not be a journal or diary. Any writing is good.

A few years ago when I was writing an article about how writing could make you happier, I contacted a well-known journalist who had written a book about his health problems and asked him how the writing process had helped him. He was so full of himself that he turned me down because I hadn't read his book. This made me feel stupid and angry, so I wrote him an e-mail pointing out that the piece wasn't about him, his ego or his book, but about the benefits of writing. It wasn't a very long e-mail and I didn't send it, but I felt a whole lot better afterwards. Five minutes – it was that easy.

So writing is good, but eventually you really want someone to answer back, and a journal won't do that. An internet chat room might talk back, but here you're talking to untrained people who may have no interest in your welfare – it is very risky. Your happiness is too important to be placed in the hands of a teenager in Tokyo, a geek in Ghent or a dropout in Darwin. In the long term, virtual communication is compounding the real problem, which is about not communicating with real people.

You also mentioned exercise

More and more GPs are beginning to prescribe it, and rightly so. Dozens of studies have shown that exercise helps mental health, improving symptoms in at least four out of five cases. It gets the body's natural pain killers – endorphins – going and it offers something new to do, new goals and sometimes even new friends. (There's more on this in the section 'Exercise: want to get back in the game?', on p. 52.)

Anything else?

Anything you enjoy that gets you out of yourself – trainspotting, double-entry book-keeping, underwater basket-weaving – may be of benefit.

Try yoga or meditation, dancing or singing. Learn relaxation techniques or have a massage or other complementary therapy. Take a walk, take a holiday or – perhaps easiest and best of all because it isn't just you who benefits – do something that helps someone else. Give a family member, friend or local charity a hand.

Last but not least, depression is in the head. You should take control of anything (alcohol or drugs, or whatever) that has a negative impact on what's going on in your head. Such indulgences *might* be the cause of the problem. (Some prescription drugs can cause depression as a side effect too.)

Can I get talking treatments on the NHS?

It can be difficult but you should ask your GP. For mild and moderate forms of depression, NICE recommends that GPs consider problem-solving therapy or counselling. NICE reckons that at least half of the people with depression or anxiety disorder could be treated successfully in this way. However, you'll be lucky to get more than six or eight sessions of help.

How do talking treatments work?

If you get it through the NHS, the talking treatment will probably be called 'counselling' or perhaps 'CBT' (cognitive behavioural therapy, which is not as daft as it sounds). It will be very focused on the specific problem – helping you to deal with relationship break-up, bereavement or job loss, for example. They don't go into the heavy stuff like your childhood, which is fine. Often just talking through the problem is all you need to see the solution.

If that doesn't work – and even if it does – you may want to go further and try to understand how you react on a deeper level. That's where therapists and self-help groups come in. They don't focus on solving a particular problem but on knowing yourself better, so that you get to see the problems on the horizon before they actually become problems.

Therapists, counsellors – whatever you want to call them – are people too, and you need to choose one you get on with. If you find one who seems to expect you to look up to them or who acts like they have all the answers and you don't, forget it. The relationship should be one between equals. In fact, it is you who has the answers. You need to talk to someone who has the skills to help you to find them.

Doesn't it take a long time?

Just as people undergoing therapy don't all look and talk like Woody Allen, so therapists don't all look and talk like Sigmund Freud. They don't bang on about your secret desire to murder your father and sleep with your mother. And you don't have to go for 20 years. Two is far more common – often a lot less.

Mid-life crisis: the best thing that ever happened to you?

Most of the e-mails to <malehealth.co.uk> are from men – no surprise there. But when we do hear from women, by far the most popular topic is the mid-life crisis – more particularly the male mid-life crisis. In most of the e-mails, he's distant, having an affair or has just quit his job. Often all three. Now, I'm not defending adultery or betrayal, but I am going to try to explain how they happen and why I think that, in the long term, the mid-life crisis may be a good thing.

First of all, it's not particularly accurate to think of it as a crisis. Crisis implies something unusual, which this isn't. In fact, the sort of psychological readjustment that this 'crisis' represents is perfectly normal. Indeed, although both can be very traumatic, what we're talking about here is no more a crisis than is puberty. Also, although it often happens in mid-life, it can occur much earlier or much later. Perhaps, to use a physical analogy, it's best seen as the psychological version of wisdom teeth – the last bit of growing up, something that usually happens much later than the other bits of growing up. As with wisdom teeth, for some people it may never come at all.

Why does mid-life crisis seem to happen so often?

Human children, like all animal babies, are socialized. They're helpless and learn by copying and imitating, but – in this vulnerable, ill-equipped state – they will make some big decisions about their future.

Taking up hobbies and sports, choosing subjects at school, beginning careers, falling in love and starting families. These all happen when we're young, at a time when we don't have any experiences of our own to draw on – only those of others to copy or imitate – and when our thinking is still coloured by the 'magical thinking' of childhood.

Although we have generally grown out of thinking that the world revolves around us, most of us in our teens and twenties still tend to think that we are protected, blessed or special in some way. (Even people who are special in some way – those with an extraordinary talent or gift – are just the same as everybody else in every other respect, and for them coming to terms with their 'ordinariness' is arguably tougher than for the rest of us.) To put it bluntly, we don't know ourselves very well when we start life's journey.

The result is that many of us wind up making choices that are not 100 per cent true to what we really are. We do things our parents want, we follow careers we think are respectable or lucrative rather than because they are our vocations, we mistake love for lust, and we form lifetime partnerships on the basis of this hormonal roller coaster which – although wonderful – can only ever be short term.

That's how adult life begins for us all and, within the space of a few short years, we suddenly find ourselves playing all these adult roles while still feeling like kids inside. We tell ourselves that we'll grow into it. If we behave like an adult, then sooner or later we'll feel like one. This can go on for a long time. Let's call this, as some do, the 'first adulthood'. The move from here into second adulthood often looks, from the outside, like the thing we're calling a mid-life crisis.

So it's not the invention of modern society?

No it is not, although it sometimes looks like it. Life used to be nasty, brutish and short, but today in the UK people live for far longer. Many have money enough to think beyond the material needs of food and shelter to intangibles such as the soul, the spirit and, yes, 'being happy'. And they have choices – many choices.

The mid-life crisis is an internal conflict between the choices you made and the choices you wish you'd made (or would have made had you known yourself better). It is a psychological conflict between the life that you're living, the roles that you're playing and what you truly are.

Second adulthood, if you can get there, is about accepting your own mortality and your own 'ordinariness'. By ordinary, I don't mean dull or uninteresting, I mean quite the opposite. What I am talking about is an understanding that you are special only in the sense that everyone else is – as a unique human being. (This is a very special specialness – a specialness that we can have no doubts about.)

Second adulthood is about knowing yourself better, knowing what makes you happy and doing it, making choices based on your own values and desires and not anyone's else's. It is not easy or always affordable, but possible. This is why some of today's retired generation are having the time of their lives.

Sounds good – how do I get it?

There's no right or wrong about this. People can experience this 'crisis' at any time. After years of singing someone else's song, Britney Spears gave every impression of going through hers at the age of 25. I reckon tennis player Andre Agassi had his just before he hit 30, when, after slumping to 140-odd in the world, he came back to establish himself as one of the best players the game has ever seen, and a very nice guy to boot.

At the same time, there are many men still in their first adulthood in their sixties or seventies. Some seem pretty happy on it – Peter Stringfellow is the sort of bloke who springs to mind. Others are in a more difficult place – showing the signs of crisis but reluctant to admit it to anyone, especially themselves.

There are even some lucky souls whose second adulthood is so close to their first that the rest of us hardly notice the transition.

The reason why the crisis occurs in mid-life for most people is that many of the triggers that can force us to start looking seriously at ourselves and our lives also happen in mid-life. Careers can stagnate and not live up to their promise. Geographical mobility can leave us further from our roots. Children become more independent. Our own parents get older, need help and – a frequent trigger – die. If that's not enough, the aches and pains in our own body serve as a daily reminder of our own mortality. Perhaps more than any other trigger, it is the grudging acceptance of the inevitability of our own

appointment with death that gives us the kick up the arse we need
– it's now or never.

OK – but why buy a red Porsche Coupe?

Initially, the things that must be done 'now or never' may appear
pretty pathetic to a non-male: buying a sports car, taking up the
latest extreme sport or sleeping with a teenager, for example. What
is going on is that we're trying to revisit the choices we made
when we were younger. (Women do this too at this time in their
lives. Those who have been at home looking after kids often find
themselves looking toward the job market and/or having affairs
themselves.)

However, if those revisited choices are still based on poor self-
knowledge, mistaken premises and inherited assumptions, then
they won't be any better than the first time and probably worse. A
man who has learned nothing may well find himself repeating the
mistake of choosing a long-term partner on the basis of immediate
sex appeal. (As a rule of thumb, the sports car is a better bet than
the trophy second wife arm candy. It's usually cheaper and you
won't, in most cases, feel the urge to impregnate it.)

The aches and pains and all they herald for the future are not
the only physical trigger of the crisis. For men, the hormone that
once got us chasing after all those first adulthood goals with such
enthusiasm is on the wane. Testosterone levels begin to fall from
the age of around 40. Replacing lost testosterone – HRT (hormone
replacement therapy) for men – might well help to prolong first
adulthood for a while but it's only delaying the inevitable. Of
course, declining testosterone is very scary – especially for men who
have always done most of their thinking with their penis. The art of
second adulthood is to see it as a great opportunity to think about
something else instead.

4

When the system goes down: how to be ill with skill

What do I do when I'm ill?

Knowing who to go to when you have a health problem will save you and your doctors' time, save the NHS money and possibly even save your life. This short guide tells you what to do and when.

When should I go to Accident and Emergency?

Would you call out roadside recovery if your car ran out of petrol? Of course not. You'd probably walk to the garage yourself or phone a friend.

Only go to A&E (Accident and Emergency) or the Casualty Department if you are bleeding, are burned, think you have broken something, poisoned or overdosed yourself, or are in severe pain. Go for the wrong reason and you'll probably spend a long time hanging around before being sent home none the better. Hundreds of men make this mistake every day.

Some people think that by ringing for an ambulance they will be seen as a priority. This is not the case. All new arrivals are assessed by a triage nurse who ensures that patients are seen in order of seriousness. Calling an ambulance when you don't need one will only annoy the very people you want to help you – the doctors and nurses – and may deny an ambulance to someone in a genuine life or death emergency.

TV programmes like *ER* can give the impression that A&E doctors are the best in their profession. This is not true. They are experts in accidents, but when it comes to, say, detecting a lump that could be cancerous, your GP is a much better bet. Look at it this way: your local panel beater may have made your dented front wing as good as new but you still wouldn't ask him to tune your engine.

Am I having a heart attack?

You're twice as likely to have a heart attack if you:

- have a waist over 37 inches (94 cm),
- smoke or
- take no exercise.

Do all three and you're a heart attack waiting to happen.

The most common symptom of a heart attack is central chest pain spreading perhaps to the arms, neck or jaw. You may also feel sick, sweaty or breathless. Less common symptoms include a 'heavy' feeling or milder discomfort in the chest, more like severe indigestion, that makes you feel generally unwell. You may feel lightheaded or dizzy.

If you think you or someone you're with is having a heart attack, get him to a hospital immediately. Chewing on an aspirin might stop further blood clots. You can dial 999 for an ambulance or 112 (the European emergency number and the international number from GSM mobiles). Make sure you know how to call the emergency services from your mobile.

OK, so I don't need A&E, but who should I see?

The best bet if there's something you're not sure about, such as a pain or a lump or a cold, sore throat or stomach upset that won't clear up, is to make an appointment to see your GP (general practitioner). It makes sense to do this because if it is serious:

- only your GP can refer you to a specialist such as a hospital consultant, physiotherapist or chiropractor, and
- only a GP's prescription will get you anything but the most basic of drugs from the pharmacist.

Your GP is probably not the only health expert at your surgery. The practice nurse, for example, can sort out holiday jabs, blood tests or other routine matters, often without an appointment. She or he can also advise you on how to use the medicines your doctor has prescribed. Some surgeries also have physiotherapists, counsellors and other specialists on site to whom the GP can refer you. Some may even have a specialist Well-Man clinic.

All GP surgeries must produce a leaflet explaining their services. Ask for one the next time you're passing. Also ask about extended opening hours. Over half of GP practices are now open in the evening or on Saturday to make it easier for working people to go.

If you're not registered with a doctor, just go into your local surgery and ask to register as a patient. If they can't take you they should point you to a practice in your area that can. If you have trouble registering with a GP, contact your local PCT (Primary Care Trust).

Symptoms to watch out for

Go to the GP if you:

- lose weight and don't know why;
- lose your appetite;
- have a sore or ulcer that does not heal;
- have a nagging cough or hoarse breathlessness that won't go away;
- cough or vomit blood;
- can't pee comfortably (e.g. if you are in pain, can't start or can't stop, want to pee a lot, or don't feel properly empty afterwards);
- have unusual discharges from any orifice (especially the penis or backside);
- have unusual growths or lumps on any part of the body;
- have a mole on the skin that is changing shape, growing, bleeding or weeping;
- have frequent changes in bowel habit – bouts of constipation or diarrhoea;
- have signs of blood – red or dark black – in your faeces;
- have regular erection problems; or
- have pain in any part of the body that won't go away or keeps coming back – this is especially important if the pain is in your chest.

None of these symptoms are particularly pleasant anyway, so it makes sense to get them sorted. They could all also be signs of something more serious that you need to get checked out.

But my GP can't see me for days

According to the Government, three-quarters of patients get to see their GP within two days, but if you're one of the unlucky ones you could call NHS Direct or try a walk-in centre in the meantime.

NHS Direct (0845 4647) is a 24/7 telephone helpline answered by a trained nurse who can advise you, in complete confidence, on what the problem might be and what to do about it. The nurse will be able to tell you who in your area will be able to help you best, which could save a lot of time. Calls are charged at local rate.

NHS walk-in centres are a kind of halfway house between your GP and NHS Direct. Found in bigger towns and cities, they're usually open from 7 a.m. to 10 p.m., and you can generally pop in without an appointment. They won't know you, which you might prefer in some cases, although without your medical history they might be less able to make a prompt diagnosis.

I don't really know how to talk to my doctor

It's not easy. Appointments are short and doctors are busy. That's why the best patient has to be a CAD.

- Come prepared;
- Ask questions;
- Discuss problems.

Try not to turn up with a list of problems, but if you do then ask about your biggest worry first. It's a mistake to mention the football-sized lump in your groin as you're backing out of the door. Talk to your GP as you would to a friend, even when he or she doesn't seem particularly interested in you. For some doctors, the impersonal approach is a way of coping in a life and death profession.

Be honest about how you feel. It's not easy to talk about problems with a complete stranger, but don't trivialize it or worry about wasting the doctor's time. Make sure that you can understand your GP's advice – if you don't know what the doctor is babbling on about, ask for an explanation.

After this appointment you won't get another chance to ask questions for a while, so make the most of it. Ask for clarification – 'What do you mean by a couple more tests?' Ask for more detail – 'How much more exercise should I take? And what sort?' Doctors are under a lot of pressure. Be realistic; they are doing their best but the truth is that medicine will always be a bit of a hit and miss affair. Don't expect instant solutions – be a patient patient.

Do I have to do what my doctor says?

No – it's your body not theirs. Generally, you'll want to follow the doctor's advice but insist on talking about it fully. Blood tests won't do you any harm, and neither will the odd X-ray or scan. These are all over in seconds.

What about the, ahem, prostate examination?

The digital rectal examination sounds very high-tech, but it's actually nothing more or less than the doctor sticking his gloved finger up your backside to feel the size of your prostate. You'll hardly notice it.

My doc wants to do a 'procedure' – what's that?

A 'procedure' can be anything that is supposed to help diagnose your problem – like a test – or treat it. Ask exactly what procedure is being proposed.

He may call it 'routine' surgery, for example, but no surgery is routine for the body on the receiving end. It's still surgery, which means there are risks, however small. Make sure you know them. Particularly important is to discuss how you'll be after the operation.

It's amazing how many men, for example, have not been told that they may have erection problems after a 'routine' prostate operation. Doctors don't seem to realize that most men do not consider no sex to be routine.

Talking of sex, what about sexually transmitted infections?

You can see your GP about absolutely anything at all, and that includes sexually transmitted diseases. However, if you'd prefer to see someone you don't know, there are specialist clinics, often in hospitals, for STIs (sexually transmitted infections).

These GUM (genitourinary medicine) clinics or STI clinics (sometimes called 'clap clinics' or 'VD clinics') offer free and confidential advice on sexual health and STIs. They can do all the tests and can, if necessary, contact previous partners anonymously. Your GP need not be told about your visit to the clinic, and you don't even need to give your name if you don't want to.

Phone first to see if you need an appointment or can just drop in. If your PCT can't tell you where your local GUM clinic is, then contact the FPA (Family Planning Association).

Can't I just buy treatments myself?

Often you can. The high street pharmacist is a good source of quick, medical advice. For many minor problems, it can be easier than going to the GP. Pharmacists can sell you over-the-counter (OTC) remedies for things like colds, sore throat, athlete's foot, dandruff or zits, and can tell you whether it's more serious than you think. If you'd prefer to speak in private rather than in front of other customers, just ask. It's normally no problem.

If you'd prefer an alternative remedy, most health food shops can offer similar advice, although they will probably not have had the professional training of a pharmacist.

What about buying over the internet?

If you have a prescription from your doctor and you want to fill it online, that is no problem. Many pharmacists have websites.

The big question is what do you do when you *haven't* got a prescription. Your best bet – and the only thing I can recommend – is to go and see your GP and get one. If you're tempted to buy prescription drugs online without a prescription, then you need to think very carefully indeed. You could wind up with the wrong drugs, counterfeit drugs, fake drugs or illegal drugs, which may be dangerous. A report by the European Alliance for Access to Safe Medicines in 2008 suggested that about two in every three pharmaceutical products sold online were fake. There's advice on how to buy safely online on <malehealth.co.uk>.

So what is the internet good for?

Used properly, the internet can be a great source of health information and support, but it needs to be handled with care. It can help you to get the most from a conversation or a consultation, but it is no substitute for a health professional and is never a substitute for real talking.

There are billions of pages out there on the world wide web and millions being added every day. In September 2008, a search for 'men's health' yielded 27,200,000 pages. How many is it up to now? For specific diseases or health problems you get even more choices. 'Cancer' throws up 249,000,000 pages, and 'smoking' 163,000,000.

Make sure you know what you're looking for and that you know how a search engine works. Put even the most trivial complaint or illness into a search engine and within a couple of clicks you'll probably find someone who has died from it. This sounds funny but it can be quite a shock. It was for me, the first time I looked up 'Hodgkin's disease'. Be prepared – the internet doesn't necessarily give you the information in the order you want it or need it.

Think about what it is precisely that you want to know and refine your search. To get the best out of a search engine, try to be specific. Use the 'advanced search' option if available. You aren't restricted to searching for individual words. You can use speech marks to search for specific phrases, for example to search for 'abdominal aortic aneurysm'. Also use + (plus) and – (minus) to narrow down your results. For example, 'smoking + "erectile dysfunction"' will retrieve items that mention the habit and its effects on your pecker. (Basically, to save you looking, the more you smoke the greater the risk – 20 a day men have nearly twice the risk of ED compared with non-smokers.)

A search for '"why does it hurt when I pee?" – Zappa' will find you the answer to a common question (answered in the question 'What are the symptoms of VD or a sexually transmitted disease?' on p. 33) avoiding references to the Frank Zappa song of the same name.

A combination of the above can be very powerful indeed, enabling pinpoint searches. For example, '"Abdominal Aortic Aneurysm" +"Dr Smith" +"Belchester Bugle"' might help you to track down a specific article in your local paper, even when the writer has the commonest of names.

Although most search engines recognize shortcuts like pluses and minuses, they don't all work in the same way, so a bit of trial and error is needed to get the best out of them. (Search engines within a particular site – rather than a global search engine like Google – can be particularly frustrating because they are frequently built on far simpler technology.) Use a different search engine to get a second opinion.

Why is the sort of information I'm searching for never top of the search list?

Despite their name, internet search engines do not actually search the internet. They search their own databases which in turn link to real websites. Search engines use programs called spiders to check these links from time to time but they are not always up to date. That's why you sometimes click on a link on a search engine to a page that is no longer there.

Spiders find new pages to add to their database by going to the pages they already know about and following the links from those pages. In other words, if a page is not linked to any other, a spider cannot find it. An unlinked site will only appear on a search engine if it has been submitted to it directly.

To decide in what order to display the pages that match your search, the search engine doesn't just count the number of times your word appears on a page, it tries to rate each page's usefulness to your search. This is a great idea in theory but very difficult in practice for a computer program to do. The result is that, at the moment, the way search engines work can be heavily weighted against sites providing good health information for its own sake.

Search engines use many different criteria to rank pages. Links is one. The theory is that if a lot of other sites are linking to a site, it must be useful. This sounds fine but may simply mean that the website has included as many links as possible – never mind the quality or relevance. Many commercial sites have long lists of recip-rocal links. Good sites choose their links more carefully. As a result they don't get so many links in return and might appear further down the search list.

Because a lot of people use the internet to buy things, search engines tend to prioritize sites which are selling something. This is not a useful criterion when you're looking for health information. You want independent information; people selling health products will provide the information that supports their products.

Commercial sites also have more time and money to try to find ways round search-engine ranking. Academic institutions like uni-versities, not-for-profit organizations and patients' groups whose information is nearly always better often don't.

So how do I know if a site is reliable?

Check out the organization or company behind it. Are *they* reliable? Many sites have an 'About us' section. If they don't have one, why not? If you don't know who is behind a site or if they're trying to sell you something, be wary. Is the site simply a shop window or part of the marketing of a product, or does it aim to provide independent information for its own sake?

Look out also for the 'HON CODE' accreditation logo. It is awarded by the Health on the Net Foundation (a not-for-profit organization attached to the United Nations) to sources of 'useful and reliable online medical and health information'. The UK Government's scheme – a seal of approval for reliable sources of information – was due to launch in 2009.

How do I talk about the thing I can't talk about?

Have you got something that you can't talk about? Something that's too embarrassing, too shameful or too bloody painful to even admit to or think about, let alone discuss? You're not alone – that I guarantee. It happens to a lot of us. The other thing I guarantee is that, whatever it is, there's someone else out there who *has* talked about it, and doing so has helped them.

Listen to Dennis: 'I just couldn't help myself. I sat alone in a one-roomed apartment and sobbed in private for months. I thought of suicide frequently.' You will understand why Dennis felt as he did when I tell you that he had just experienced what is probably a man's greatest nightmare: having his penis cut off. Following cancer of the penis – which is very, very rare – Dennis's was amputated and a new one created using a skin graft from his leg.

This is Dennis later: 'If only someone had told me that talking about my new penis openly would help, I'd have done it far sooner. I hope that writing this on <malehealth.co.uk> will encourage and help other men to open up and talk.'

I've interviewed and talked to dozens of men who have had to deal with difficult things, and if I had a quid for every one of them who has said 'I wish somebody had told me it would help to talk about it', I could buy a football club.

Listen to these two lads talking the morning after the night before: '"I wet myself last night," my friend Pete said. Handing him a coffee and two Nurofen, I agreed that the previous evening had been a laugh. "No," he said. "I really did." Then he broke down in tears.'

That's from an article on <malehealth.co.uk> about urinary incontinence – peeing when you don't want to. Danny Farthing, who wrote the article, had no idea about his friend's problem. Why? Well, as Pete put it, 'Mate, I'd rather tell someone I can't get it up than admit I wet myself.' You might well agree with him, but the article had a happy ending. There are several organizations out there helping people with urinary incontinence. Pete contacted one and got the help he needed.

In fact, there are support groups out there for nearly every condition and concern you can think of, and more. Paruresis, for example, is a condition that most of us have suffered from at some time. Also known as 'shy bladder syndrome', it's the inability to pee in public. You know the story, a crowded public toilet and you can't pressurize yourself, but for some people it happens all the time and it can be soul-destroying. You literally cannot go out.

'What sort of man are you if you can't even piss? Your self-esteem plummets,' one man told me. Another, Ian, said: 'This must be one of the most secretive afflictions going.' Perhaps, but the UKPT (UK Paruresis Trust) can help. Ian's life was turned around by a UKPT workshop. 'Beforehand I was terrified,' he said. 'I wondered if they were a bunch of nutters. As I checked into the hotel I was trying to work out who else couldn't pee. But the weekend worked. Afterwards I felt absolutely liberated. If someone had told me that after the workshop I'd have been able to pee with someone standing next to me I wouldn't have believed them.'

It's a great example of how patients' groups, self-help groups and voluntary organizations can make a real difference to people with a health problem – and quickly.

One of the most frequently read articles on <malehealth.co.uk> has the headline, 'I never felt confident about getting married, have never got involved with anyone in that way, and never will.' It's about hypospadias, a birth defect that affects about one man in 125 in which the penis doesn't develop properly and the opening is in the wrong place. One reason why the page is so popular is that it is one of the very few on the internet about this condition.

Many people got in touch – both parents of children with the condition and men who had grown up with it. Most of the men had never spoken about it before. I put them in touch with Wilf, who had written the original article. Together, they set up the UK's first self-help group for men with hypospadias.

'It has been extraordinary,' said Wilf when I interviewed him about the overwhelming response to his article. 'It just seems to go on and on. We're reaching a lot of men who haven't talked about this much before. They're discovering that they're not alone. There are common elements to the stories of most of the men who have contacted me. They had something that was supposedly "dealt with" while they were young. They didn't really know what it was and their parents were unable to talk about it. They grew up not knowing and unable to find further information.' The support group will plug that gap.

A lot of people criticize the internet because, they say, it means we don't talk to each other any more. I disagree. I think it's actually made it easier for us to talk to each other about the things that matter. It's far easier to send an e-mail than it is to turn up at a meeting or even make a phone call. It's not as good as real talking, but doing one thing can make it easier to do the next thing. Little steps are easier to take than big ones.

If you think you're alone, you're not. Have a look on the internet and if you can't find anyone you want to talk to, try <malehealth .co.uk>.

I admit that I think talking is 'a good thing' because it helped me, but I challenge you to come up with a single personal, emotional or health problem that won't be helped by talking about it, especially with someone else who has had the same or a similar experience. It may only help a little but it will help.

Talking can help violent men, murderers, wife beaters and sex offenders alike – and prevent other men from becoming like them. Talking can help men who have been abused, tortured or terrorized. If it can do all these things, it can almost certainly help you. Just don't open your heart on television.

If you're still not convinced, there are more men talking about difficult subjects throughout this book.

How can talking really help?

It might not straight away. At first, especially if you're talking about something that has been part of your life for a long time, talking may feel like a waste of time. This applies regardless of who you're talking to – a mate, your partner, a self-help group or even a professional therapist.

The reason is obvious if you think about it. At first, you'll be talking about stuff you've talked about a lot before – the things that have brought you to where you are. All familiar material, but stick with it. One day you will say something that you've never consciously thought before and then it will start getting interesting.

If you're in a self-help group it may even take a while before you want to say anything at all. That's fine too. Listening to people talking about something that seems to have nothing to do with you can trigger off real insights into yourself.

Talking might not always be easy. A good listener will ask questions that are directly relevant to what you're saying. They will make you think and make you work. That too can be pretty uncomfortable. If you've been living with something for a long time, all those stories that you've told yourself a hundred times before will suddenly be under the microscope. Talking around them will bring out all the little flaws and self-deceptions in them.

When this starts happening it's very easy to decide that it is all too difficult and you want to stop. Eventually, though, all the crap in your head comes back and frequently, because you're older, in a more gruesome form.

One day you may realize that talking is just less painful than not talking and waiting for all your demons to come back again. It's like that moment when you decide to turn and confront a bully. It might hurt but it might stop him doing it again, and it's certainly better than living in constant fear that he's going to be waiting around the next street corner.

How do I handle a health problem?

Having a health problem changes you. It affects you physically and affects your mood. Even something small like a cold or a sore knee. Now, obviously you don't want to bang on about it, but learning how to accept the little health problems will help you to deal better with the bigger ones if they come along. Don't pretend it's not happening and be honest with yourself about the difference it is making to your life.

This is why it's worth working on your mental health. If you're feeling reasonably happy about yourself and who you are, you'll be able to cope with pretty much any physical health problem life throws at you. If you're angry or unhappy, a touch of cold or flu can knock you for six, to say nothing of a serious health problem.

I want to find out more about my health problem

When first diagnosed, some people want to know everything about their problem; others want to know nothing at all. Neither is right nor wrong; it depends on the person and on the problem. However, sooner or later you'll probably want to know more. When you do, use your research to quiz your doctors more thoroughly, and always discuss what you've learned with them before acting on your findings – you don't want to do something that will reduce the effectiveness of the treatment they're providing.

Talk to people at your clinic. The doctor may be too busy for an in-depth chat but what about your nurses, pharmacist or physiotherapist? Other patients can be helpful too. They may not be experts in the disease (although some will probably think they are), but they know about living with it and can sometimes provide a surprising amount of support.

Talk to specialist organizations. There are hundreds of charities and voluntary organizations dealing with particular health problems, and there may well be one for you. They provide specialist information and the chance to talk to experts and other people who have experienced the disease. They may run self-help groups or offer counselling and advice. You can find organizations online.

Also, read. Books are the best way to build up a picture of your disease because you can read them at your own pace, whenever and wherever you want, and return to them as often as you like. Make sure you get a book aimed at patients rather than at doctors, and check that the author can actually write well – not all doctors can. For this reason you might be better off choosing books written by health journalists. Check the publication date and the dates of the research quoted; general books won't date too much, but if a book offers more detail on a particular subject you'll want it to be as up-to-date as possible.

Read newspapers and magazines too, but be critical. News, by definition, tends to be about extremes, so health stories are often about crises, rare or unusual medical experiences, or research break-throughs. Sometimes quite everyday stuff can be overplayed by the media; even if it is a genuine breakthrough it will take several years for the research to have any impact on patient care.

If you've been diagnosed with a health problem, it's even more important to use the internet with care. Try to visit websites that you can trust, such as those recommended by health professionals, other quality sites such as <malehealth.co.uk> or those hosted by respected organizations. This is a better approach than just typing the name of your disease into a search engine. Join lists and discussion groups only when you're beginning to understand your illness and what it means.

Is it worth trying complementary therapies?

The same advice applies as for the internet. Yes, it's worth investigating but be careful and make sure you know what you're getting into.

The term 'complementary therapy' covers a broad range of treatments. While some such as chiropractic, acupuncture and osteopathy are now generally accepted by the medical establishment, it is very sceptical about others such as homeopathy and aromatherapy.

Complementary therapies work in different ways. Some offer potions or pills, some involve the manipulation or massage of the body, and others call for new skills to be learned or different life-styles to be adopted. Some claim to work by faith alone, but they all put you and your views at the centre of the process, and this alone can be a big boost.

Sometimes a therapy might claim to cure a disease, but more often they ease symptoms or simply make you feel better in yourself. The one thing all approaches have in common is that someone, somewhere, thinks they work.

When research shows that people benefit from complementary therapies, some doctors dismiss it as all in the patient's mind, or the 'placebo effect'. They might be right, but why should you care? Most people just want to feel better. Leave the scientists to worry about the how and the why. The placebo effect only emphasizes something I've been banging on about all the way through this book – the importance of your mental attitude in health and healing.

The best way to find a therapist is through recommendation, preferably from your doctor or another health professional whom you respect. But you can also ask fellow patients or friends, check out local health and leisure centres, or look at notice boards in doctors, pharmacists or health food shops.

Check out your therapist – however highly recommended, you need to be sure that he or she is right for you. There's not much regulation of health claims, so be sceptical. Fortunately, many complementary therapies have regulatory bodies that should be able to provide a list of registered practitioners in your area, but check what inclusion on the list means. Does it indicate particular qualifications or experience, or only that a membership fee has been paid? Beware of any therapist approaching you and offering an instant cure – as a rule of thumb, the more therapists promise the less they're likely to deliver.

Quiz your therapist before committing yourself. What exactly does he do? How long has he been doing it? How did she start? What training has she had? Where did he train and for how long? What professional bodies does she belong to? How long will each session take? How long will the whole programme take? What sort of benefits might you expect to see, and when? How much will it cost?

A key question is, is he insured? Few insurers will insure unqualified practitioners. No decent therapist will mind the questioning. Theirs is a person-centred approach, so it will be important to them that you feel comfortable.

Check you can afford it. Discuss costs with your GP. The range of therapies to which a doctor can refer patients is increasing all the time. Some voluntary organizations may be able to help. There may be sessions at a local authority leisure centre or other council facility.

If you don't like the treatment, the therapist or the way he explains himself – some of the theories are very hard to believe – then quit. No decent therapist will object, so don't be bullied into staying. On the other hand, don't give up if results aren't imme-diate. Discuss your concerns with the therapist.

Get into it. To benefit from complementary therapy you need to be both open-minded and self-centred. You need to let yourself go without giving up responsibility for your health to someone else.

How do I make the best possible recovery?

If you follow the advice provided in this book, you won't go far wrong.

Don't try to do too much too soon. Once you're on the mend, it's easy to assume that everything is back to normal. It isn't. Recovery is gradual not instant. Don't go back to work too early after flu, don't play sport too soon after an injury, and don't expect to have your strength back as soon as your cancer is in remission. Through impatience you could relapse, and that is very depressing.

For more serious conditions, it can be harder to let it go. If you've accepted your condition, your disease will have become a part of your life. Once you recover, it will become a much smaller part, and that transition can be difficult.

One minute the doctors are worried about you and the nurses are caring for you, the next they hardly notice when you arrive for a check-up. This can be especially tough if you have been in hospital for a while. This is why many patients seek counselling or therapy at the end of an illness.

I've got a long-term problem that won't go away

Living with an LTC (long-term condition) or a disability may be the biggest challenge of your life, but – as with all big challenges – the feeling when you come out the other side is priceless. Some disabled men will tell you that their disability is one of the best things that has happened to them, that they have developed as people and understand themselves and others better. Even those who don't feel so comfortable about their disability will say it has made them stronger.

Disability is a perfectly normal thing. If you think about it, we are all only temporarily non-disabled. At some time in the future, whether through age, illness or accident, we will all become more or less disabled.

Over the years I've interviewed a lot of men living with a variety of long-term or chronic conditions. When the Men's Health Forum made LTCs the theme of Men's Health Week in 2007, I collected together their tips and advice. These are summarized below.

Live in the present

An LTC will change your life. You will be a different person afterwards and it's better for your long-term physical and mental well-being to recognize this than to pretend that nothing has happened. This may involve you in grieving for some aspect of your old self, your old body or your old life that has gone. It's fine to be sad. It's good, it's normal, and – like with any other bereavement – with time comes acceptance. It's important not to fight this.

Learn about yourself

When coming to terms with an LTC, you'll find yourself asking a lot of pretty basic – and tough – questions about yourself and your life. This is good. You'll come to know and understand yourself better, which will make you stronger, more confident and better able to make decisions about your own happiness. Because greater self-knowledge involves facing up to yourself as you really are, it can involve looking under some unpleasant stones. Therapy or counselling can often be a big help here.

Meet people like you

Thanks in no small measure to the internet, there are now voluntary groups, organizations, forums and chat rooms for people with every LTC you can think of, and more. It's an important part of not denying your condition but recognizing it as part of you.

When you're talking to other people under these circumstances, try to see the similarities between your life and those of others. By seeing the similarities we have with others, it is far easier to learn from them and about ourselves.

Your condition also gives you something very important in common with the others in the group, which can enable you to get to know each other more quickly and more deeply than in everyday life. It can result in your making some excellent long-term friends who really know you.

You are even more unique!

You are possibly the only person with your LTC among your family and friends and work colleagues. That means that you bring a unique insight into life and work that is born out of living with your LTC every day.

More and more smart employers are embracing difference. They know that firms who always employ the same kind of people always come up with the same kind of solutions, and that's simply not good enough in today's competitive market. Original, imaginative people who can think outside the box – and people with LTCs are often all of these because they have to be – are increasingly sought after.

Don't become a junior doctor

Take an interest in the medical developments that affect your LTC but don't become obsessed with reading everything you can in every journal and on every website. You need to take what you read in the mainstream media with a pinch of salt, and for some websites you'll need a whole salt cellar.

Don't place all your hopes on a medical breakthrough and forget the word 'cure'. Obviously, you'll want to take your doctor's appointments seriously, but you're a person not a medical condition. Live your life. Let the doctors do their job and you do yours.

5

Inside the operating system: A–Z of other user-serviceable parts

The human body is always delivered fully assembled – much to the relief of new mothers. If it came in a furniture-style flat pack, however, it would have a contents list containing the following parts.

Here's a whistle-stop tour of the key remaining parts of the body and how to keep them in top working order. It is worth skimming through even if it's only to find out what to do about the common cold (p. 119) and how to get a decent night's sleep (p. 112).

Armpit

What does it do?

Smell.

What's good for it?

Washing and using a deodorant (sweat is odourless until bacteria gets to it). If you're allergic to regular types, try natural deodorants or one without aluminium.

Arteries

What do they do?

Carry blood from the heart. The largest, the aorta, emerges from the left ventricle of the heart.

What can go wrong?

See the section 'The heart' (Chapter 2). Blood clots (an embolism or thrombosis) can also block arteries. Several thousand British men lose their lives every year to abdominal aortic aneurysm, a blockage in the aorta. It is becoming more common but can easily be detected using an ultrasound scan. In 2008, the Government promised to introduce screening for men over 65.

What's good for them?

See heart, on p. 16. A small amount of aspirin can thin the blood, reducing risks of blockage, but only use this technique under medical supervision.

Favourite food

Spinach (helps regulate blood pressure).

Bladder

What does it do?

Needs to be emptied whenever you're more than a mile from a public lavatory. It is connected to the kidneys by two tubes; the average male bladder holds over half a litre.

What can go wrong?

Cystitis, bladder stones (from a low protein diet) and occasionally bladder cancer (more common in men than women). Feeling the need to empty your bladder a lot or difficulties doing so could be the sign of a prostate problem (see the section on the prostate on p. 28).

What's good for it?

Some say exercising the urethral muscle (just pretend you're trying not to pee) between the bladder and urethra can improve erections and orgasm quality. Feels weird though, doesn't it?

Favourite food

Watercress – can break up bladder stones.

Bones

What do they do?

Stop your body from collapsing sack-like in an undignified heap. There are 206 of them in your skeleton.

What can go wrong?

Osteoarthritis, nutritional disorders (called rickets in kids or osteo-malacia in adults) and hormonal disorders such as osteoporosis.

(Osteoporosis does not just affect women: one in five men over the age of 50 will break a bone because of osteoporosis.)

What's good for them?

Calcium and vitamin D make strong bones, but it's largely done in childhood, so supplements won't help now. However, exercise strengthens bones and sunlight helps vitamin D absorption.

Favourite food

Oats (good for bones and connective tissue) and figs (good source of calcium).

Bowel

What is it?

The rest of the digestive system – the bit that isn't your stomach. It is made up of the small and large intestines. Curiously enough, the small one measures 6.5 m while the large one which surrounds it is just 1.5 m.

What can go wrong?

From food poisoning to exotic diseases like cholera and typhoid to cancer by way of inflammatory conditions such as colitis and Crohn's disease.

What's good for it?

Most of the nasties can be avoided by keeping up your fibre intake (from fruit and veg and beans, grains and pulses). For constipation, try a bulking agent like Fybogel. For the opposite problems, try Immodium (and keep fluid intake up).

Bleeding from the behind affects about one in ten people and is usually not too serious, with haemorrhoids (or piles) the most likely offender. Don't be shy, though. See your doctor promptly if your stools contain blood or look oily and black, or if problems recur frequently.

Bowel cancer is the third biggest cancer killer of men, but 90 per cent of cases can be treated if caught early. If you're over 50 ask your GP about bowel cancer screening – an easy test you do at home – or call the NHS Bowel Cancer Screening programme helpline (0800 707 60 60).

Favourite food

Cabbage – it detoxifies the stomach and colon.

Butt

What does it do?

Keeps you upright. It's thanks to your behind – or more specifically the gluteal muscles it masks – that you're not on all fours like other apes. Surveys also show that a man's bottom is, in the view of most females, the second most interesting part of his anatomy. (And the answer to the question you're about to ask is the eyes.)

What can go wrong?

Not a lot – a misplaced drawing pin perhaps. Itchy backside can be caused by, among other things, poor hygiene, tight non-cotton underwear, biological washing powders or perfumed fabric softeners. Try dabbing on carbolic lotion (1 in 100 strength) twice a day.

Your behind can give you warning signs of bowel problems. (See the section on 'Bowel', above.)

What's good for it?

Squats (legs slightly apart and making as if to sit down) and lunges (making as if to kneel on one knee without actually making contact) are good butt-firming exercises.

Ears

What do they do?

Process sounds, maintain balance and look ridiculous in photos.

What can go wrong?

The ear is pretty well protected, although infections are not uncommon. Tumours in the ear are rare – we don't know yet if mobile phone use will see them increase. Like the eyes, the ears become less efficient with age, particularly with regard to phrases like 'it's your round' and 'haven't you had enough pie?'

What's good for them?

Avoiding thrash metal concerts (nothing to do with your ears – just avoid them).

Eyes

What do they do?

Provide a 3D multicoloured view with perfect perspective using 137 million light-sensitive cells for the total real-life experience.

What can go wrong?

Our eyes have evolved to be effective at distance – for hunting. Modern life, with its screens and books, is conducted in close-up so the eyes get tired (needing rest and exercise) or deteriorate (needing glasses).

What's good for them?

An eye test every two years and, if you're prescribed glasses, wearing them. (If you use computer screens or displays in your work your employer should pay for an eye test.) If you prefer contacts, accept that the risk of conjunctivitis and other infections is increased and follow the cleaning guidelines. Look away from your computer screen every so often (yes, gazing out of windows is good for you!).

When working with sparks and splinters or playing sports like squash and swimming, wear the appropriate protective goggles. Sunglasses should conform to European Standard BS EN 1836.

To exercise your eyes, try frequent blinking and ten minutes of 'palming' a day (simply covering the eye with the palm to exclude all light). Another exercise is to slowly move your splayed hand in front of your eyes so they focus close up on the fingers and in long distance on the spaces between.

What's good for keeping eyes shut?

See box 'Zzzzz: tips for getting some shut-eye'.

Zzzzz: tips for getting some shut-eye

- Keep regular(ish) hours and a regular bedtime routine which helps you wind down (a warm shower and a dull book rather than three hours of serious poker and a Red Bull).
- Avoid stimulants before bed, including exercise, caffeine, fags, booze and heavy meals (a light snack and/or warm but dull drink is OK as you don't want to go to bed hungry).
- Use the bed for sleep (and sex) – laptops and TV are a no-no. Reading is fine but stick to something that will make you doze off, not a racy thriller.
- Avoid bright light before bed – dim the lights in the rooms you're in before bed as well as the bedroom.
- Don't clock watch or stress – if you can't sleep get up and do something boring.
- Make sure the bedroom isn't too hot – it should be a degree or so colder than the rest of your home.
- Try sleeping alone if you usually sleep with someone (or *vice versa*!).

Favourite food

Carrots or blueberries – it's the betacarotene, see.

Feet and toes

What do they do?

More work than any other part of your body, probably. Good for over 100,000 miles with only basic maintenance, these 26 brilliantly put together bones, which both support the body's weight and propel it forward, are one of the planet's most efficient – and green – means of locomotion.

What can go wrong?

Mostly irritants, such as bunions, corns and blisters. Also a common site for gout – a curable form of arthritis.

What's good for them?

Footwear with half an inch between the tip of your longest toe of your biggest foot and the end of the shoe. To prevent blisters, the heel must be firmly in place. Avoid slip-ons – they're usually too tight – and buy shoes in the afternoon when feet are at their biggest.

Get the right footwear for your chosen sport. A bit of Vaseline goes a long way toward preventing blisters.

For sweaty feet choose easy breathing shoes such as sandals and use a talc. Bathe ingrowing toe nails in warm, salt water and see a GP or chiropodist. Treat athlete's foot (itchy, dry red skin) with antifungal cream or powder and a verruca (brownish growth with pepper pot appearance) with gel. Both are available over the counter in the pharmacist's. See a GP or chiropodist if they don't clear.

Hair

What does it do?

Fall out.

What can go wrong?

Too much falls out – 20 per cent of men are balding by 30 and about 60 per cent by 50. It still bothers some men, but there's no link between baldness and anything serious such as heart disease.

What's good for it?

The best way to avoid baldness is to be castrated before puberty. If you don't fancy this, a testosterone friendly diet like that described on p. 27 (see the question on 'Can you boost testosterone levels naturally?') might help. This is not because baldness is related to excessive testosterone – sorry – but because of the way your body processes the hormone and turns it into new ones. Avoid stress – it diverts blood from the less essential areas like the scalp to the muscles and brain – and brush your barnet frequently.

Drugs to treat baldness might help you to keep your existing hair a little longer but they won't do much to restore what you've lost. It's easier, less stressful and less expensive to go bald gracefully.

Favourite food

Lemon (for treating greasy hair).

Hands and fingers

What do they do?

Pretty much anything you want. The hands – with their incredible opposable thumbs – are an evolutionary masterpiece and probably the main reason it's us running the show and not the baboons. More flexible than a wallet full of credit cards, fingers are good for 25 million bends in a lifetime.

What can go wrong?

Warts, boils and repetitive strain injury (computer games mean that even young children are getting RSI).

What's good for them?

Rubbing palms with astringent oils like geranium or cypress might help if you have sweaty palms. Even easier, just brush back your hair before shaking someone's hand.

Three-quarters of warts will disappear within a few months but persistent offenders can be zapped with a salicylic acid solution from the chemist. See your GP if it doesn't work.

Treat chapped or dry hands with a handcream.

Tips for avoiding RSI are given on p. 68 (see the question 'What can I do myself to make my own working environment healthier?').

Joints

What are they there for?

To enable the body to do the many things it does. Types: ball and socket (shoulders); hinge (elbow); pivot (neck); and ellipsoidal (wrist). Cartilage acts as shock absorber between two bones, which are held in position by ligaments.

What can go wrong?

Cartilage damage, sprains, torn ligaments, osteoarthritis (wear and tear) and rheumatoid arthritis (an immune system disease).

What's good for them?

See knees (below) and feet and toes (above). Exercise joints by stretching them through their full range of movement (particularly important as you get older).

Favourite food
Eggs (but not fried).

Kidney
What does it do?
Filter out waste and water from blood and food. The two kidneys weigh about 170 g each and filter about 1,500 litres of blood (that's over 2,500 pints) daily.

What can go wrong?
From kidney stones to damage from diabetes or (very rarely) tumours, the kidney is not the most robust organ in the body. Luckily, only one is strictly needed.

What's good for it?
Drinking plenty of water.

Favourite food
Beetroot can clear kidney stones.

Knees
What are they for?
To get down on at that momentous moment in every man's life.

What can go wrong?
When you run you put several times your body weight through your knees, which is why half of professional footballers have arthritis, many while they are still young.

What's good for them?
Keeping weight down, running on grass rather than concrete and swimming. Do a range of movement exercises – straightening your legs without bearing weight keeps knees flexible. Here are a couple of good exercises to strengthen the muscles above the knee and reduce wear on the joint.

- Lie with a rolled up towel under the knee, straighten one knee raising the heel. Hold and relax. Repeat frequently and with light weights if you want.

- Stand or lie flat with legs straight, pull your feet toward you and tighten the muscles above the knee. Hold for three seconds and relax. This can be done pretty much anywhere – standing in a queue, for example.
- Place a pillow between your thighs and squeeze it. Again this can be done lying or standing.

Favourite food

Nettle tea – good for gout and arthritis.

Liver

What does it do?

Process and store nutrients, plasma and glycogen. It is the body's largest internal organ, weighing up to 1.5 kg.

What can go wrong?

Up to 75 per cent of the liver can be destroyed before it stops working, but it still needs to be treated with care to avoid hepatitis, cirrhosis and cancer.

What's good for it?

Alcohol is the biggest cause of liver disease. See p. 46 (section 'Alcohol: when does serious drinking become dangerous drinking?').

Favourite food

Broccoli – it stimulates the liver, among other benefits.

Lungs

What are they?

A pair of sponges. They take in oxygen, pass it into the blood stream through 600 million tiny air pockets called alveoli and expel carbon dioxide. I mean tiny – each alveolus is smaller than a grain of salt.

We inhale about five litres of air each minute. For a professional footballer in mid-game, it's nearer 200 litres.

What can go wrong?

Quite a lot unfortunately – asthma, bronchitis, pneumonia and lung cancer, the biggest cancer killer of men.

What's good for them?

Packing in the fags – the earlier you started and the more you smoke, the bigger the risk of cancer and pretty much all lung diseases. Regular exercise (20 minutes three times a week, which leaves you breathless) will improve your lungs' performance.

In tandem with the heart, the lungs form the body's cardiovascular system – its engine – so all the stuff that's good for your heart (see the section on 'The heart' on p. 16) will also benefit your lungs.

Muscles

What do they do?

Enable the body to move. There are about 600 of them. About 40 per cent of the male body weight is muscle. Muscle fibres, which are thinner than the hairs on your head, are made up of proteins.

What can go wrong?

Pulls, tears, cramps and so on – usually the result of over-exercising or not warming up properly beforehand. Although normal body temperature is 36.5–37.5 degrees C, muscles function best at 38.5 degrees C.

What's good for them?

Using them. Do strengthening and stretching exercises. Wrap up after exercise and drink plenty of fluids. There's more on exercise on p. 52 (see the section entitled 'Exercise: want to get back in the game?'). Heat can relax the muscles whereas ice reduces spasm.

Nails

What do they do?

Grow. Formed by dead tissue growing from a living base, nails grow at about a millimetre every ten days.

What can go wrong?

Breaks and similar tragedies. Nails are a good early warning sign of more serious problems (see box 'Fingernail warning signs'). During surgery, for example, the anaesthetist will use your fingernails to check whether you're getting enough oxygen.

Fingernail warning signs

- White, pale or very weak nails can be a sign of iron or vitamin deficiency or a sign of possible anaemia, or a liver or kidney problem.
- Backward bending nails can be caused by a lack of iron. Eat more green veg and nuts.
- White flecks are usually the result of a knock.
- Blue nails represent poor circulation resulting from cold or perhaps a heart or lung problem.
- Grooves across nails. You're probably recovering from a serious illness a few months ago, because illness can slow nail growth and cause grooving.
- See your GP if any of these persist.

What's good for them?

An oval finish rather than a straight or pointy one, which reduces breakages, apparently. Don't file immediately after washing as the nails are too soft and may split – major manicure mayhem.

Favourite food

Fresh vegetables – nutritional deficiencies often show up in the nails.

Nerves

What do they do?

Carry information around the body. There are 12 pairs of cranial nerves (linking to the brain) and 31 pairs of spinal nerves.

What can go wrong?

Nutritional disorders, injuries, viruses and autoimmune diseases can all damage the nerves, while many, many things can get on them.

What's good for them?

Never watching programmes featuring Anne Robinson or Jeremy Clarkson and keeping an eye on the booze and vitamin B levels. Treat a trapped nerve with ice and professional manipulation.

Favourite food

Brown rice can calm the nerves.

Nose

What does it do?

It is the entrance to the main freeway into Lung City and home to 20 types of odour-sensitive receptors – some 20 million in total. It is also excellent for sticking into other people's business.

What can go wrong?

Frequent irritants like breaks, bleeds or colds, rather than anything serious. The nose has won a design award for its unique ability to harbour mucus.

What's good for it?

See the box 'How do you treat the common cold?'

How do you treat the common cold?

We're living in a golden age for colds, says Professor Ron Eccles, Head of the Common Cold Centre at Cardiff University. It's mainly because we're travelling more in more crowded cities. Cold and flu viruses are usually caught by:

- breathing in infected water droplets in the air from someone else's sneezes or coughs, or
- by touching the eyes or nose after hands have picked up the virus from contaminated objects like telephones, towels or door handles.

So when colds are around, wash your hands frequently and don't touch your face with your hand (use a tissue). As we get older, our respiratory systems become weaker and colds and flu can be more serious. For many people the final cause of death is actually a cold.

So, Ron, have you found a cure for the common cold yet?
We already have a very good cure – the human immune system. It's a matter of trying to avoid the infections in the first place and then helping the immune system to control them if you catch one.

How do you avoid them?
The only guaranteed way is to avoid all human contact. Failing

that, keep your immune system in top form. You do that by maintaining your general health with exercise, rest and a balanced diet. Insufficient sleep will have a major impact because the immune system restores itself during sleep.

What else can help?
- Zinc is very important to the immune system. Because the main sources of zinc are red meat and seafood, vegetarians may need to consider a zinc supplement. With that possible exception, supplements are not necessary for most people.
- Echinacea does appear to be useful in influencing the immune system and can control infection, but it's not black and white when it comes to colds.
- I wouldn't take vitamin C to prevent a cold, but at the very first sign of one a couple of grams of vitamin C may help as an anti-oxidant.
- The sort of substances we used in the past to preserve food, such as garlic and onion, are also helpful because they have natural antiviral properties. Garlic is nature's own antibiotic. A hot soup or hot curry can encourage mucus secretion.
- Mucus is the immune system's first line of defence, so you want to get that going. Make sure you don't drink too much because alcohol encourages nasal congestion. Take plenty of hot fluids instead – the nasal mucous membranes need to be well hydrated to block infection effectively.
- Listen to your body. If it tells you you're tired, go to bed. Your immune system is asking for some help. Give it some.

Wrap up warm?
Yes. Flu and cold viruses can only reproduce at 32 degrees C or below, which is below human body temperature, so if you keep your nose warm with a scarf or balaclava the virus can't replicate itself. A hot bath or sauna will work too.

What about the flu jab?
I'd recommend a flu jab in September for anyone over 65 and for younger people who are at increased risk as a result of asthma, heart problems, diabetes or a less effective immune system. If you're fit and healthy it may be better to have flu. Some people won't even notice. Just like a cold, flu ranges from mild to severe.

Can a sinus infection after a cold be worse than the cold itself?
Yes. You need to take an oral decongestant containing pseudo-ephedrine, but it's not suitable for everyone, especially those with high blood pressure, so you need to discuss it with your doctor first.

Menthol and eucalyptus vapours are helpful too – just a couple of drops in a bowl of boiling water. They're warming and have a mild antibacterial effect too.

Favourite food

Chicken curry – clears the airways and stimulates snot production.

Skin

What does it do?

Keep all the gooey stuff inside. Skin is about 5 mm thick and constitutes one-twelfth of your body weight, making it your heaviest organ.

What can go wrong?

Every minute nearly 40,000 cells fall from the skin (that's 4 kg a year). When this goes wrong, dry skin, eczema or psoriasis can result. Rates of skin cancer are doubling every ten years.

What's good for it?

A balanced diet, vitamins and a little sunlight. Also drink plenty of water, and use a pH-balanced soap and a decent moisturizer.

Sun helps the body to create vitamin D, keeping bones strong and preventing osteoporosis. For this, it needs direct sun (up to 20 minutes with no sunscreen) every day, including cloudy ones. This amount of sun will not cause skin cancer, but too long in the sun unprotected can. Don't burn and avoid the hottest part of the day. The two best skin cancer protectors are called a hat and T-shirt. Make sure you get your anti-oxidants (selenium and vitamins C and E) plus betacarotene (in carrots) and lycopene (tomatoes). Choose a natural sunscreen without oxybenzone for the bits you can't cover.

Favourite food

Fresh fruit (yes, Mum was right).

Spine

What does it do?

Support the entire skeleton and house the spinal cord (a tube of nerves that with the brain make up the central nervous system).

The functional requirements of the spine – that it is both flexible and weight bearing – make it a designer's nightmare. Evolution hasn't done too bad a job, but with 33 cylindrical bones (vertebrae) stacked one on top of the other to form the spine and more than 150 joints in this area, it's perhaps no surprise that back pain is the UK's second biggest cause of sick leave, leading to five million lost working days a year.

What can go wrong?

Back problems run in families but work can make a big difference too. Occupations with high accident levels or repetitive physical tasks are risky. Less obvious hazards are train driving, washing up and checkout operating. Motorists clocking over 25,000 miles a year are seven times more likely to have back pain than low mileage drivers.

What's good for it?

Stretching it. Set up your desk and car seat properly so that you're not over-reaching and the lower back is supported. Stretch. Lift properly (from the knees not the back), don't over-use the phone and, rather than using a single heavy bag, carry loads evenly in a rucksack or two smaller bags. Stretch. Follow the tips for avoiding RSI on p. 68 (see the section entitled 'What can I do myself to make my own working environment healthier?'). Stretch.

In bed you should ideally be lying so that neither the neck nor spine are bent. One pillow and a firm mattress is the most likely combination to achieve this. The budget solution is a firm board between mattress and bed base.

Alexander Technique, chiropractic, osteopathy, yoga or massage all help back problems. If you are in pain, keep moving. Even though some doctors still recommend it, taking to your bed can make things worse (damn!). And, if we haven't mentioned it already, stretch. Finally, however much you love them, lay off the high heels. Cushioned soles are best, for example trainers.

Favourite food

Fatty fish such as salmon.

Stomach

What does it do?

Process all that junk you put in your mouth. The digestive system is about 9 m long, although the stomach forms only about 20 cm of this.

What can go wrong?

From indigestion and the like to inflammation (gastroenteritis), ulcers and tumours (stomach cancer kills about 13,000 a year).

What's good for it?

Plenty of fibre in the diet (see the section on bowel, p. 109). Ask your pharmacist about a remedy like Gaviscon for indigestion and heartburn.

Favourite food

Ginger – prevents nausea or travel sickness, eases indigestion and, as the docs delicately put it, 'quells flatulence'.

Teeth

What are they for?

To make you go to the dentist. Adults have 32 of them.

What can go wrong?

Decay both of teeth and gums. As you get older you're more likely to lose teeth through untreated gum disease than through decay. Bleeding is an early sign of gum disease. Gum disease may be an early sign of heart disease. Receding gums expose the roots of teeth, which can become sensitive to hot and cold. A toothpaste for sensitive teeth will help.

What's good for them?

Brushing for five minutes each day. Hold your brush like a pen and brush away from the gum using short horizontal movements with a soft to medium bristle. Buy a new brush every three months. Brush or floss bleeding areas. If they persist see your dentist (and see one every year, anyway). Dentists can also treat bad breath if a two-stage mouthwash from the pharmacist doesn't work.

Favourite food

Parsley freshens the breath while turnip eaten raw helps clean teeth and aid digestion. (This must be why Baldrick in *Blackadder* has such fine gnashers.)

Throat

What does it do?

Become sore immediately an unpleasant task is suggested.

What can go wrong?

Sore throat is usually a symptom of cold, flu or too much shouting (see box 'How do you treat the common cold?', on p. 119).

What's good for it?

Gargling salt water.

Favourite food

Grapefruit helps with throat infections.

6

DIY health check

Your car gets one regularly but what about you? No, not a speeding ticket – an MOT.

You've read the book. So how are you doing? Your body's once-over doesn't require any spanners and needn't cost a penny. For most blokes, most private health checks are a waste of time and money. They offer nothing that you and your GP can't offer. If you're worried about the results of these five home tests, see your GP.

Are you fit?

Pulse

Check your pulse. Place the finger of one hand on the thumb side of the tendons running through the opposite wrist. You should be able to feel the radial artery pumping. Count the beats over four 15-second periods and add them up. This is your resting pulse – a good guide to the heart's efficiency.

Joggers and other fitness enthusiasts will get very excited about resting pulse and try to get it as low as possible. Lance Armstrong was their hero. At his peak, the cyclist reportedly had a resting pulse nearer 30 than 40. A slug's is nearer 90.

Recovery rate

Check your recovery rate. Step on and off a step for three minutes (average a step every three seconds) and rest for 30 seconds before taking your pulse again. See Table 2 for a guide to recovery rates.

If you're in or close to the unfit range, you need to think about whether you're taking enough exercise. See the section entitled 'Exercise: want to get back in the game?' on p. 52.

Table 2 Recovery rates

Age	Resting	After exercise	Resting	After exercise	Resting	After exercise
Teens/20s	59 or less	75 or less	60–85	76–101	86+	102+
30s	63 or less	79 or less	64–85	80–103	86+	104+
40s	65 or less	81 or less	66–89	82–105	90+	106+
50s plus	67 or less	83 or less	68–89	84–107	90+	108+
	Very fit		*Average*		*Unfit*	

If you're aged over 30, obese or have an existing health problem, check with your GP before starting an exercise programme.

Are you fat?

Work out your body mass index using the formula given in box 'What's your BMI (body mass index)?' on p. 39. If your BMI is over 25, you are overweight. Read the section 'Eating: want weight loss without great loss?' on p. 37. If it is more than 30 or under 20, see your GP. If you have been losing weight for no apparent reason, it may be a sign of something serious – see your GP.

A simpler guide than BMI is your waist measurement – over 37 inches and you're getting fat. Again, read the section on eating on p. 37.

Examine the hardware

Check yourself all over for five things:

- moles changing shape;
- unexplained lumps;
- swelling or itching;
- a cough that won't go away; and
- blood where it shouldn't be (in saliva when you spit or in crap).

If you find these talk to your GP.

Monitor performance

Complete the checklist 'How long have I got?' in Chapter 1. Do it regularly. In which direction is your life expectancy going?

Check your blood pressure

Ideally, your GP should do this but you can buy home testers. BP – as they say in the hospital dramas – is given as two figures. The first is when the heart is contracting (systolic) and the second when it is resting (diastolic). In other words, the diastolic figure is effectively your resting pulse. 120/70 would be fine for a young man. Once the systolic starts getting up toward 140 and/or the diastolic to 90, you need to talk to your GP. There's more on blood pressure on p. 20.

7

A little summary

Good health is not a big deal. It's about little changes. This book is about those little changes – little changes to diet or routine or attitude, a little more exercise, and a little bit of thought about why you do the things you do.

Most of what you read about health is misleading. Much of it actually has little to do with health. Health is not about how many calories you eat or the number of bench presses you can do. It's not even about whether you even know what a bench press is. (Is it like a trouser press?) Health is not something you can count. As I said in the section 'Work: the twenty-first century's biggest threat to health?' in Chapter 3, nothing that counts in life can be counted. I mentioned imagination, fun, love and laughter in that chapter. I should finish by adding self-awareness to that list. (Some people call it emotional intelligence.) It's probably the most important of all as far as good health is concerned.

There's a thin line between a couple of pints to unwind and a drink problem. There's a thin line between a little lump and a cancer. There's a thin line between a healthy obsession and a dangerous addiction. There's a thin line between being cool and level headed and being detached and lonely. There's a thin line, as Chrissie Hynde of the Pretenders once gorgeously pointed out, between love and hate. Self-awareness is knowing which side of the line you're on.

In this book there's also much talk about talk. The most important person to learn to talk to is yourself.

If you're able to step back from how you feel, look at your actions, look at your emotions and be honest with yourself – you can see clearly which side of the line you're on. To get from one side of a thin line to the other, you don't need to go very far, and that's where all those little changes in this book can help.

Useful addresses

Action on Smoking and Health (ASH)
First Floor, 144–145 Shoreditch High Street
London E1 6JE
Tel.: 020 7739 5902
Website: www.ash.org.uk

Addictions
Website: www.addictions.co.uk

Alcohol Concern
64 Leman Street
London E1 8EU
Tel.: 020 7264 0510
Website: www.alcoholconcern .org.uk

Alcoholics Anonymous
PO Box 1
10 Toft Green
York YO1 7ND
National Helpline: 0845 769 7555
Website: www.alcoholics-anonymous.org.uk

Alzheimer's Society
Devon House
58 St Katharine's Way
London E1W 1JX
Tel.: 020 7423 3500

Beating Addictions
Website: www.beatingaddictions .co.uk

Blood Pressure Association
60 Cranmer Terrace
London SW17 0QS
Tel.: 0845 241 0976
Heart health information line:
08450 70 80 70

Website: www.bpassoc.org.uk

British Heart Foundation
Greater London House
180 Hampstead Road
London NW1 7AW
Tel.: 0845 241 0976
Website www.bhf.org.uk

British Nutrition Foundation
High Holborn House
52–54 High Holborn
London WC1V 6RQ
Tel.: 020 7404 6504
Website: www.nutrition.org.uk

Cancerbackup
Freephone Helpline: 0808 800 1234
(8 a.m. to 8 p.m., Monday to Friday)
Website: www.cancerbackup.org.uk

See also **Macmillan Cancer Support**, with whom it merged in April 2008.

Depression Alliance
212 Spitfire Studios
63–71 Collier Street
London N1 9BE
Information Pack Request Line:
0845 123 23 20
Website: www.depressionalliance .org.uk

Fpa (formerly the **Family Planning Association**)
50 Featherstone Street
London EC1Y 8QU
Tel.: 020 7608 5240
Helpline: 0845 122 8690 (9 a.m. to 6 p.m., Monday to Friday)
Website: www.fpa.org.uk

Infertility Network UK
Charter House
43 St Leonards Road
Bexhill
East Sussex TN40 1JA
Tel.: 0800 808 7464
Website: www.infertilitynetworkuk
.com

**International Stress Management
Association**
PO Box 491
Bradley Stoke
Bristol BS34 9AH
Tel.: 0117 969 72384

Lucy Faithfull Foundation
Freephone: 0808 1000 900
Website: http://lucyfaithfull.org

Macmillan Cancer Support (now
part of **Cancerbackup)**
89 Albert Embankment
London SE1 7UQ
Tel.: 020 7840 7840
Website: www.macmillan.org.uk

Male Health
Website: www.malehealth.co.uk
Provides information on various
aspects of male health.

Men's Health Forum
Website: www.menshealthforum
.co.uk
A UK male health policy site, which
also runs the site <www.malehealth
.co.uk> giving a wide range of health
information for men.

NHS Direct
Helpline for advice: 0845 46 47
Website: www.nhsdirect.nhs.uk

Orchid Cancer Appeal
St Bartholomew's Hospital

London EC1A 7BE
Website: www.orchid-cancer.org.uk
(for men with prostate or testicular
cancer)

Prostate Cancer Charity
First Floor, Cambridge House
100 Cambridge Grove
London W6 0LE
Tel.: 020 8222 7622 (general)
Helpline: 0800 074 8383 (10 a.m.
to 4 p.m., Monday to Friday)

Quitline (for advice and
information on stopping smoking)
Tel.: 0800 00 22 00
Website: www.quit.org.uk

Relate
Herbert Gray College
Little Church Street
Rugby
Warwickshire CV21 3AP
Tel.: 0300 100 1234
Website: www.relate.org.uk

Samaritans
Tel.: 08457 90 90 90 (24 hrs)
Website: www.samaritans.org

Sexual Dysfunction Association
(formerly **Impotence Association**)
Suite 301, Emblem House
London Bridge Hospital
Tooley Street
London SE1 2PR
Helpline: 0870 7743571 (10 a.m. to 4
p.m., Monday, Wednesday, Friday)
Website: www.sda.uk.net/

WorkSMART
Website: www.worksmart.org.uk
A site set up by the Trades Unions
Congress (TUC) to provide
information and guidance for
today's working people.

Further reading

Real Health for Men (2002) by Peter Baker (easy to read, thoroughly researched and wide ranging. It is out of print but well worth seeking out in libraries and secondhand bookshops.)

The Man Manual (2007) by Dr Ian Banks (the best-selling men's health book, in the style of the classic Haynes car maintenance manuals.)

The Complete Book of Men's Health (1999) by Dr Sarah Brewer (the original men's health handbook and still one of the best. It is also out of print but worth seeking out.)

Men's Health – How To Do It (2007) edited by David Conrad and Alan White (a basic handbook for health professionals and policy-makers trying to communicate with men about their health.)

The best starting point for further reading on the web are the sites run by the Men's Health Forum and the NHS. See p. 130 for more details.

Index

A&E (Accident and Emergency) 89
accidents 7
addiction 4, 71–7
adolescence 10
alcohol 4, 5, 46–52
alcohol units 47–8, 50
alcoholism 51–52, 74–5
anger 4, 79
anti-depressants 81
anti-oxidants 45
aorta 107
armpit 107
arteries 20, 107
aspirin 108

back problems 122–3
backside 110
baldness 113
bladder 108
blood 12, 18, 34, 107
blood pressure 20, 22, 49, 127
body mass index (BMI) 39
bones 108
bowel 109
bowel cancer 109
brain 12–16, 48
brain size 15
brain tumours 15

cancer 6, 49
cereal 45
chips 46
chromosomes 8
colds 119–21
concussion 13
condoms 35
complementary therapies 102–3
complementary therapists 103
core strength 56

dementia 15
deodorants 107
depression 77–85
diet 18, 37–8

disability 104
Disability Discrimination Act 67
drugs, illegal 4, 15, 27

ears (and hearing) 110
eating 39–41
eating disorders 75–6
electromagnetism 68–9
embarrassing problems 97–100
erection problems 24–5
evolution 41, 69
exercise 4, 5, 13, 18, 19, 52–63, 83
eyes 111

fats 42
feet 112
fish 4
free radicals 45
friendship 4, 80
fruit and veg 3, 5, 43–4

gambling 76–7
genes 6
GP (general practitioner) 4, 90–3, 126
gyms 62–3

hair 113
hands 114
hangover 51
happiness 8
health and safety 67
heart 16–20, 57
heart attack 6, 8, 90
heart disease 6, 20
heart rate, maximum and minimum 61
hypospadias 98–9

incontinence 98
internet 26, 34, 94–7, 99, 102, 105

joints 114

kidney 115

knees 115

lifestyle 6–8
liver 48–9, 116
long-term health conditions 104–6
lungs 116

masturbation 31–2
meat 4, 42
memory 16
mid-life crisis 85–8
minerals 28, 43–4
muscles 117

nails 117–18
nerves 118
neurotransmitters 13
NHS Direct 92
NHS walk-in clinics 92
nose 119

omega-3 fatty acids 45
orgasm 23
over-exercise 62
over-work 65

pacemaker 19
paruresis 98
patients' organizations 101, 105
penis 20–8, 97
penis size 21, 23
pharmacists 94
placebo effect 103
plants 69
plaque 20
pornography 31, 74
premature death 1
prostate 28–30, 93
prostate cancer 29
prostitution 32
pulse 17, 125–26

reading 4, 82, 101
recovery from illness 104
repetitive strain injury (RSI) 68
respiratory disease 7

risk 6–7, 9, 50
running 56

St John's Wort 82
salt 41
self-awareness 128
sex 4, 30–5, 49,
sexual offences 32–3
sexuality 31
sexually transmitted infections (STIs)
    33–4, 93
skin 121
sick building syndrome 69–70
sleep 4, 36, 112
smoking 4, 5, 25, 117
sperm 22, 23, 27
spine 122
sports drinks 59
sports injuries 57–8
sports shoes 59–60
statistics, understanding 47
stomach 123
stress 4, 18, 66, 70–1
stretching 53, 114, 115, 117, 122
stroke 12
sugar 41
suicide 77–8
sunlight 4, 121
swimming 56

talking 80, 97–100
talking therapies 81, 84–5
teeth 123–4
testicular cancer 28
testosterone 10, 25, 26–7, 88
throat 124

vasectomy 35
vitamins 28, 41–4, 109

walking 4, 56
warming up 53–5, 58–9
wealth 8
weight 18, 37–9, 57, 126
work 4, 37, 63–71, 73–4
writing 82–3